CONTENTS

NOTE:
Apart from those who, by virtue of their offices, are readily
identifiable and those others who have also given specific
permission for their real names to be used, most of the persons
named in the book have, although they are real persons, been
given pseudonyms in order to preserve their privacy.

FOREWORD

This book is a testimony to personal courage and determination supported by a strong Christian faith. The author's vivid writing and frankness enable us to share intimately in her moments of joy and of occasional despair during the acute and rehabilitation stages of the illness which began in the very hospital in which she had worked as a trained social worker and member of the health care team.

Although it is now more than six years since her cerebral haemorrhage, the description of events and reactions are remarkably detailed and therefore all the more telling. Her initial inability to communicate, in spite of clarity of thought, led her to go over and over in her own mind what she wanted to say. Her pre-operative review of her life, her 'last' letter to her parents and her description of the times when she wanted to communicate but could not are particularly poignant – at the time she wanted to write a diary for the interest of her attendants and of the public but nothing would come in writing let alone in speech. What frustration!

As an account of an illness and of the stages of recovery, this book will grip the reader. But there is more to it than that – the author shows that professionals are very often insufficiently taught to explore their own reactions to different situations and she has sound opinions on deficiencies in education and in training programmes. She rightly criticizes the attitude that staff are all-knowing and that patients are – or should be – thankfully all-accepting! She describes with great sensitivity the inter-relationship between patients and staff of all categories and her own perceptions of the reasons lying behind different attitudes. But all this is a two-way process and we are naturally seeing it from one side – this is where the book is intended to provoke thought.

The author, while full of praise for many aspects of the care she was given and for those who gave it, is frankly critical of certain features of the health service and of present-day society. The scene is set in Edinburgh, but the same criticisms would apply elsewhere and it is the author's frank personal assessment of places, people and things that stops the reader in his tracks and shakes him out of any complacency he may have. The same incidents and attitudes seen through different eyes might give quite different impressions and lead to different conclusions. Perhaps some patients improve as a result of having something to complain about other than their own illness; it can take them out of themselves.

I have known the author for four years and have seen the book develop. I am sure that the last thing she would want would be any feeling of pity for what she has had to go through; nor would she necessarily want us to agree with all that she says; rather she would want us to learn from her experience not only of the sustaining force of her faith but of the importance for each of us to look afresh at our attitudes to other people both in health care and in neighbourliness and in attitudes to disability.

Archie Duncan
Professor Emeritus of Medical Education
University of Edinburgh

CHAPTER ONE

Haemorrhage

Sunlight was streaming through my office window, the light catching particles of dust in the air and making them sparkle like minute diamonds. The Out-Patients' Department beyond my office door was quiet, almost deserted. The warmth and stillness made the atmosphere soporific. It was too near lunch-time to begin anything new. I gazed at the poster of Loch Faskally on my office wall; so like the Salzkammergut. Only the week before I had returned from a brilliant holiday there, staying with Austrian friends.

Daydreaming, I recaptured the day of my departure. Harry, his parents and younger sister had all come to the airport to say goodbye. On the steps of the Trident I turned, eagerly scanning the sea of faces for the little group I had come to love so well. There they were; I smiled and waved, my happiness tinged with sadness. For the first time in my life, I had had a holiday from which I had no wish to return. My mind flitted back a year to the summer of '73, when we had first met at the Dunedin International Folk Dance Festival in Edinburgh. I had been in charge of accommodation, and guide for the Austrian Siebenbürger team. Egon, the leader of the group, was quiet yet powerful. His English was non-existent and my German not much better, but his son, Harry, was bi-lingual. We had become good friends and the year's correspondence had resulted in this visit.

From my seat on the plane I peered through the window to see if I could find the family amongst the now indistinguishable row of tiny figures. I have never been afraid of flying; on the contrary I enjoy it, particularly the thrust of the engines during take-off and the slow climb away from the ground. I have inherited my father's enthusiasm for flying, although not his accompanying mathematical genius! He is

1

Reliability Engineer to Hawker Siddeley Dynamics Engineering and I had enjoyed several summer vacations as a student working amongst his colleagues. I had captured a little of their enthusiasm.

On this flight, I had become gradually aware that all was not well with the aircraft. Suddenly we flew into a violent Alpine storm. The little girl sitting next to me became very frightened. I tried to distract her fear by talking to her about how storms and lightning develop. She had become so interested, as her mother and I explained why we were being buffeted about in the strong up and down draughts inside the cloud, that she forgot to be afraid. All three of us watched jagged arrows of lightning pass inside our wing span, within feet of the plane. I had been fascinated and completely unafraid, accepting the storm as the answer to my premonition. In fact it wasn't: I was sitting on an internal time-bomb.

By the time we landed at Heathrow, collected our luggage and cleared Customs, we were three hours late. As I emerged from Customs my parents were waiting. In one of her flashes of extra-sensory perception, my mother had been very worried. We both talked too fast.

'You didn't expect to land, did you?' she asked bluntly.

'No,' I admitted with equal directness.

I felt as though I had been granted a reprieve. After an all-too-brief day with my parents, I was on my way back to Edinburgh. They would be beginning their own holiday the following week, travelling with their caravan to the north of Scotland, visiting me briefly on their way south.

I returned to my work as social worker to the Radiotherapy Unit delighted to find that nothing dramatic had happened in my absence: new admissions, nothing more. The social work and nursing staffs who inquired about my holiday caught the enthusiasm in my voice, but I had little for my work. In social work if you don't have your heart in it, you only do half a job. I had decided that today, Monday, would be different. Did I feel different? Certainly this morning more of the usual energy had pervaded my work, more of the customary enthusiasm. On the way to lunch I met Sue, the younger sister of one of my old university friends. She was an SRN, studying here for her midwifery qualifications. It was providential that day. We chose our salads and settled to the serious business of eating and exchanging news.

Suddenly, I felt a strange and ominous trickling inside the back of my head. I remembered vividly when I had felt the same sensation before and what it heralded. Should I say anything in case I inexplicably collapsed? Was it my imagination? No, it was too clear for that; a distinct sticky trickling. I stretched my neck, absurdly trying to escape the leakage inside my head. What if I was wrong? It would cause turmoil and I would end up with a very red face. But if my guess was right and I hadn't spoken, Sue would get a fright when I collapsed and it would take Casualty a long time, probably too long, to discover the origin of the problem. So I said, as nonchalantly as possible: 'Don't worry, but I think I'm having another cerebral haemorrhage. If I am, please get me to DSN3.'

Then I collapsed. I cannot remember whether it was on to the table or the floor.

'What a ridiculous colour to collapse in!' I thought. 'Why ever did you come to work today in a white dress?'

I answered my own rhetorical question.

'Because you wanted today to be different. Well, nothing will ever be the same again!'

Around me there was chaos and great scraping of chairs.

'I'm sorry. I didn't mean to cause all this bother.'

I heard Sue's voice, the edge of panic well under control, calling instructions to the doctors having lunch.

'Good old Sue, she didn't ask for this.'

Her frightened face flashed in front of me and was gone. I thought protectively of my surgeon; they would be trying to find him now. I hoped they would break the news gently, unhurriedly, not bluntly, 'Kristine Gibbs has had another cerebral haemorrhage.'

The first haemorrhage had been in January '67, my first year at Edinburgh University. At school I had been afraid of not getting the high entrance qualifications demanded by Edinburgh and consequently had worked myself hard. During my upper sixth year at an English grammar school, I averaged about twenty-five hours' homework each week. I'd survived without cracking, maintaining throughout half-a-dozen outside interests. When I went into a totally new environment at university, I had decided to limit my outside interests to country dancing, the Savoy Opera Group for whom I was wardrobe mistress, occasional theatres and concerts.

All had gone well for the first term and I had gone happily home for the Christmas vacation, complete with tales of my new boy-friend. I was still feeling insecure academically. The one area of life in which I knew I shone was Scottish Country Dancing. By Christmas I had been the youngest member of the University's New Scotland demonstration team for some time. My father had come up to Edinburgh on business at the end of January. After dinner on Burns' Night, he had returned to England full of stories about how happy I was.

On the last Saturday in January auditions were held to choose the Scottish Universities' Country Dancing Team to go to Russia at Easter for three weeks. There were dancers from the other Scottish universities competing. The results were announced at the end; I was through. Later that same evening I was in a friend's room in Hall, cutting out lace for a blouse for a forthcoming ball. Suddenly my head felt very strange and my hands seemed not to belong to each other. It had been a cerebral haemorrhage. Now, seven years later, it had happened again.

Memories of the previous occasion flashed across my mind. The kindness of the ambulance men as they lifted me on to the stretcher; its dangerous slope as they carried me down three flights of stairs because the lift was too small for the stretcher; the race across the city with siren going. Memories were patchy as I slipped in and out of consciousness. On that occasion it had taken time, several lumbar punctures, four angiograms and a lumbar air to locate the site of the haemorrhage. When finally traced, the knot of capillaries that had burst had been so close to the centre of my brain and beginning to heal, that it had been safer to leave it to seal naturally. So I had kept my long hair. In the intervening years it had been cut and was now merely shoulder-length. Not so much to lose if I survived as far as an operation. I gave a wry smile. People get anxious about the most ridiculous things!

I remembered from 1967 my surgeon saying:

4

'I doubt whether you could survive another one.'

I looked at the prospect quite matter of factly. I was twenty-six: sooner or later I was going to die, probably sooner. Not in the least perturbed, I wondered why. Suddenly I remembered my experience the previous week on the plane and my lack of fear. That had been good planning on the Lord's part to give me the experience before I would need it. I smiled, sharing a little of His infinite foresight. I felt as though I was adrift in a vast ocean, but quite calm and totally unafraid. It was too late for fear. My only concern was about how my surgeon, parents and Harry would cope with the news.

'Please Lord, calmly, maturely; don't leave them until it's all over.' So floating somewhere between the Snack Bar and the main hospital corridor, I decided that I would do my best to survive positively for as long as possible, and that I would not give up.

The previous haemorrhage had paralysed the right side of my body below eye-level, but within a week the effects had disappeared above my waist. Only my right leg was left in spasm, paralysed and very weak. I had fiercely fought a move by my surgeon and physiotherapists to have a calliper made; you could not dance with a calliper. I had visualised the calliper merely encouraging the muscles to deteriorate. There had been a note of desperation in my struggle. The calliper would have been the final defeat, the signal to relinquish the fight as lost. I could try to fight people, but not rigid iron-work.

After four weeks my surgeon had been convinced that I could manage without the dreaded calliper. Against one of the leading surgeons in the country, the physiotherapists didn't stand a chance. With much hard work from my dancing teacher, who was also a doctor, and myself, a return to dancing was achieved. In 1969 I went with the New Scotland Team to dance in an International Festival at Neustadt in Schleswig-Holstein. I knew I was the worst dancer in the team, compensating for my weak right foot with my strong left one and that all the apparent bounce in my right ankle was produced by bending my right knee. I had developed the art until it was scarcely noticeable under a long white dress.

Occasionally people stared, but I had danced for Scotland. Flushed with personal triumph, I smiled when people looked askance at my weak right foot and thought, 'If only you knew!'

Gradually other things replaced the need to dance. I graduated in 1970, and, following a decision made when I was about fifteen, had taken the Edinburgh post-graduate Diploma in Social Work. As I became increasingly absorbed in my work, dancing ceased to be so much a necessity, and more like the icing on top of the cake. My work became my primary form of self-expression. I had first worked for a children's agency in Edinburgh for whom I had become a student supervisor. Early in 1974, I started to think of spreading my wings. A post to which I felt I had much to contribute was advertised at one of the city's general hospitals. Even better, it included work with students. It was the sort of hospital post in which I had visualised myself at the climax of my career. The only problem was whether I was ready for such a post now. I had decided to apply and leave the planning to God. If I didn't apply, I should never know. I had submitted an application, ready for Him to say 'No, too soon' – and was appointed. So it was in mid-April that I had started on the Radiotherapy Unit, and was soon seeing positive results from my work.

Now slowly I became aware of light, brilliant sunshine and an upward slope; the approach of the Department of Surgical Neurology. I struggled into semi-consciousness, my mind accepting the realization with pleasure before black unconsciousness descended again. The only reason why I survived the haemorrhage to begin the fight at all was because of my warning, the availability of my surgeon at the time of my collapse and the fact that he was able to inject a semi-sealing drug directly into my brain.

CHAPTER TWO

'She could be paralysed . . .'

It all began for my parents late in the afternoon on Wednesday, 28th August. They were driving quietly along near Largs when a small car dashed past, the driver flagging them down. A pretty blond woman came running back towards them. 'Have you a daughter Kristine, in Edinburgh, and is your name Gibbs?' she asked breathlessly. They answered 'Yes' to both questions, unknown fear rising inside them. The young woman continued: 'Did you not hear the news? An S.O.S. has just come over the radio for you. They read out your registration number and you were in front of me. Your daughter is critically ill. Follow me and I will take you to the Police Station.'

There they phoned my surgeon who explained that he did not think that this haemorrhage was quite as severe as the previous one, and said: 'Come at once.' On the journey to Edinburgh, both spoke little, each busy with their own thoughts, aware of the silent support of the other. The day began to fade and watching the clouds drift past, my mother wondered whether they would arrive too late. She remembered the previous time when they had been given the same instructions. Then they had been at home in Hertfordshire and the quickest way had been to fly. They had managed to get two stand-by seats and had sat holding hands trying to support each other, wondering what would greet them at the other end. It had been my mother's first experience of flying. This time they would know the hospital and had a good knowledge of the Department of Surgical Neurology. They left the car and caravan in the department car park, remembering it from seven years previously.

Both were worrying about breaking the news to my brother. The last time he had still been at school and in an exam year,

7

but had insisted on staying at home alone, trying to study. Since then he had graduated from Leicester University, and was now working on Bio-Physics research there. Still worrying about contacting him as they walked up the path, my mother automatically looked up to the ward area. There was a tall, lone figure, bowed and forlorn silhouetted in the window. It looked just like Andrew, but it couldn't be. The figure turned and waved: it was Andy!

The Police had contacted him from the address in my diary. He had driven up and, as my flat-mate was on holiday, was staying in my flat. In my father's absence he had assumed responsibility and given permission for any necessary action to be taken. Now they were all taken in together to see me. My mother told me later:

'I shall never forget that moment; you looked like a little brown shadow, so frail, as if you were already far away. We gently kissed your cheek, and your eyelids fluttered. You were lying on your side with your hands clasped by your face. One hand patted the pillow softly as you whispered: "Hello, I'm sorry I'm not very well just now." '

As they stood quietly beside me, my mother noticed that there were straps on my wrists and asked if I was going to theatre. The nurse explained that I had to be tube-fed through my nose, and I objected so violently that if not tied down throughout, I would simply pull the tube out. My mother was given permission to remove them. After a while my parents went to see Sister, who said that they were welcome to stay if they wished but as I had just begun to turn the corner, advised them to get some sleep. They could visit or phone in the night if they wished, and my surgeon would like to see them in the morning.

They took their caravan to its usual site in Edinburgh, and arranged to park as near the gate as possible. Andy would be in the flat, and should any message come from the hospital during the night, he would drive out to the caravan park with the warning. The previous day, urgently travelling north in his sports car, just north of Duns he had hit an oil slick on the road. Automatically he put his skid training into practice. The car spun drastically and ended up facing the other way, but still on four wheels. It had taken the tread completely off one of his tyres and reduced the life expectancy of the others considerably.

Now he was planning a possible midnight race across the city, knowing the stresses under which he would be driving. As he left my parents, he said kindly but sternly to my mother:

'It's happened, Mum. You can't undo it. You've got to learn to live with it.' So typical of my brother; no wasted words. My parents slept fitfully, clinging to each other in the darkness for comfort. Every time a car turned in at the gate, they were both immediately alert, my mother sitting up in fright. Morning found them heavy-eyed and fearful.

They kept their appointment with my surgeon, finding him little altered in the intervening seven years and just as forthright. He expressed his sorrow about the second haemorrhage and blamed himself for not operating on the previous occasion. He explained that since it had occurred in the hospital itself and he had been close at hand, he had been able to get a semi-sealing drug directly into my brain. It was a last chance. He told them quite openly that even while he tried it, he didn't hold out much hope for my survival. Everyone was practically holding their breath. My parents assured him that they felt his previous decision had been right, borne out by seven happy, abundantly active, dynamic years.

The semi-sealing drug had worked. In a week to ten days I should be strong enough to withstand angiograms. He felt sure that the bleed was in the same area, but they had to be certain. This time there would definitely have to be an operation. He told them frankly all the things which could happen:

'She could be paralysed in both legs, both arms, lose her speech and half the sight of her right eye, to any depth and in any combination.' He noticed my mother's horror, and she expressed her fear for my legs. His reply, blunt and practical as ever, was:

'A social worker can go about her job in a wheelchair, but not if she cannot speak.'

My mother knew this only too well, but in her mind she was seeing me dancing, smiling in the sunshine at the Harpenden Highland Games, and practising my speciality which

9

had been a solo highland dance called 'Blue Bonnets'. Her face showed her thoughts. My surgeon said:

'Cheer up! We may have her running up and down stairs yet!'

Relatives are not regarded as an anxious nuisance on that unit, and are encouraged to come in whenever they want to, or need reassurance. My parents were told:

'Come in and just stay by her bed. If she flickers her eyelids and sees you there, it all helps' and, 'If you cannot sleep for worrying, just phone in and talk.'

They never did, because there was only one external telephone on the ward and they always felt that while they were phoning simply for support, they might be blocking a really urgent call; but they appreciated it and were grateful for the understanding.

By Sunday 31st August, I was strong enough to take solid food again. My brother painstakingly cut my lunch into tiny pieces, giving a running commentary to my mother on technique for future reference. I watched his every move, talking with my eyes. With great effort I could open my mouth a little, and all meals had to be fed through this narrow aperture. As any exertion might create problems, I was not allowed to sit up, so there was the added difficulty of feeding me flat on my back.

That afternoon my brother had to return to England. He had been in Edinburgh nearly a week and had to return to his work. We were not to meet again until Christmas. After that day, while I still needed to be fed, a rota was developed for feeding me: staff at breakfast, father at lunch and my mother at suppertime. This was rather unfortunate, because it meant that she always saw me at my poorest, most exhausted state.

There was also a further problem, although the staff did not realize it at the time. I had no realization of the present; no memory, no recall. Apparently, or so I was teased by the staff, at first I spoke approximately half the time in German! Later this was confirmed by the only friend who, as a research physicist connected with the hospital, was allowed to see me at the beginning and who was greeted aggressively when he arrived:

10

'Are you Harry?'

'No, Harry's in Austria!'

Slowly I became conscious of where I was, recognizing it immediately, but not associating the scene with the present at all. I just assumed that I was dreaming and imagined that my brain was somehow producing recalls of 1967. Gradually I faced the possibility that it might be real and came to the unfortunate conclusion that it was not a dream. I don't remember feeling worried or frightened, just tired, for I knew then that if I survived it would be a marathon fight. On the one hand, the easiest way out would be to die, get it over with and go home. Yet, on the other, I was enormously curious about what was going to happen, and how I would cope if I survived.

Some kind person had given me an enormous bar of very exotic soap. In examining it for the maker's name, I began to realize that I had been conscious but unaware for more than a few days. The name was completely worn away and illegible. How long had I been there? In the circumstances, I could understand my not remembering a couple of days. Yet with only one person using it, a bar of soap that large does not get worn smooth in days; it takes weeks. The realization shocked me. How long had I been unconscious? What had I missed? I discovered that it was now early September. Painstakingly, I weeded through the vast empty blackness, trying to retrieve incidents which would hold the past fortnight together. Several times each day, during nursing rounds for blood pressure and temperature, the nurses would check my reality-awareness, questioning my name, where I was, the date, day, month and year. At first I accepted it as part of the routine, but when it continued check after check, day after day, when I knew that I was giving correct answers, I wanted desperately to rebel, to answer questions about my location with something ridiculous like Timbuctu or Vladivostock. Knowing that it was not the nurses' fault, I held my tongue, gritted my teeth and instead gave pedantically correct answers, hoping that eventually the message would get through.

My parents had permission to bring me in peaches, one of my favourite fruits. What joy to sink my teeth into the succulent, juicy fruit! The realization that every one might be the last heightened the experience. I laughed at my mother's amazement the first time I held out my hand for my daily peach and just bit into the fruit. Their bloom, colour and flavour became a major topic of conversation. It was my parents' unconscious way of sharing the fact that I might not be alive much longer. I tried as gently as I could to let them know that I did not mind talking about death. I upbraided myself, knowing that I could and should face death head on. But I was uncertain whether my parents could face my death if it came, and so I tried to protect them by not expressing to them the full meaning of their unintentional messages.

CHAPTER THREE

Survival is a Matter of Will

In mid-September my father had to go on a one day business
trip to England. My mother walked to the hospital, discovering when she arrived that I had had a severe set-back. I
was lying pillowless, flat down, and in severe pain. My brain
was producing extra cerebral fluid as a cushion to protect the
damaged area. From being well-orientated in space and time,
I was having periods of disorientation caused by pain. Shortly
before the end of visiting time, the young resident houseman
came into my room and announced cheerfully that he wished
to give me a lumbar puncture. My parents helped him wheel
my bed through to the treatment room and, as visiting time
was ending, they said goodnight. I could sense my mother's
emotion and called to her at the door. She turned round,
anxiety written across her face. I smiled and signalled to her
that I would be all right. The heavy door swung to and they
were gone. We all talked as the doctor and the two nurses
gowned and scrubbed up. The machine switched on, they
turned their attention to me, baring the lumbar area of my
spine from which the fluid was to be taken. I turned on to
my side.

Then, with the resident explaining every move in advance,
he curled me into a fetal position. I was glad of his gentle
thoughtfulness and the running commentary, wondering how
many frightened patients he had reassured. He disinfected
my back; the brown liquid was very cold. I was then given
a mild local anaesthetic to ease the puncture. I could feel him
delicately counting the vertebrae, carefully checking each pro-
jection until he was certain, and then the insertion of the
needle into the liquid surrounding and protecting the spinal
cord. I was curious about the extraction, because during the
actual puncture, with a long hollow needle projecting in to

13

the spinal column in the small of my back, movement was absurd.

When the necessary two phials of spinal fluid had been removed and it was over, the doctor held them up for me to see. They were quite pinkish with blood. Gradually, on subsequent occasions when he repeated this gesture, they became clearer as the cerebral fluid replaced itself, until they were pale cream and quite transparent. On this occasion, as after all lumbar punctures, I had to spend several hours flat on my back, so flat that I couldn't even have a pillow, thus reducing an unbearable headache to manageable proportions.

By this time X-ray plates had been taken of my brain and plans were being made for the operation. However, this incident changed things. My parents were told that there would be another delay, whilst I regained strength. They remembered the statistics of 20 – 30 days for a subsequent bleed and, having been told that another haemorrhage could be fatal, they were thoroughly bewildered.

One day my mother came into my room to find me sitting in a chair, very tired but pleased with myself. The triumph had been about the chair, but the effort of sitting upright had been exhausting. I did not dare make a move by myself in case I fell, knowing that the least thing might set off another haemorrhage. I could not reach my bell, and no passing nurses had been alerted by my gentle signals. So I just sat. It was a great relief when my mother arrived, although I was anxious not to alarm her by appearing as tired as I really was. She fetched the Sister, and the two of them helped me back to bed, where I collapsed.

Although I accepted the first eye-check for intracranial pressure quite willingly, I became increasingly disgruntled with repeated examinations that evening. If I was going to die, I'd die anyway. If God intended me to live, I would live no matter what.

The following day my surgeon explained that the plans had been readjusted. There was still to be the operation; but not yet. My body had responded, as it had done seven years before, and I had improved considerably in the third week. It had been decided to build up my resistance as much as possible for the operation. Simply to keep me in bed could

14

cause clots, which could prove just as disastrous as another haemorrhage. Therefore I should be encouraged to get up for short periods. I looked at my surgeon quizzically. I needed no encouragement to get up, but I wondered whether he fully realized that there is an optimum time for such operations psychologically, as well as physically. Or, if he did, whether he realized just how close I was to my optimum.

Sometime later I mentioned to my parents that my holiday films should be back from processing, and pressed for them to be brought into the hospital. At first the medical and nursing staff were reluctant to permit it, and it seemed as though they would not allow it before the operation. However, I did not know whether I should be alive after it and was forced to take things into my own hands, making it quite plain that denying my request would have greater long-term risks to my health than the short-term one of my getting over-excited. Finally they capitulated on the understanding that my parents only brought in one box of slides each day, and that I was not to be overtired.

On the first evening my father arrived with a portable screen, which was a great surprise and delight. The film show was enjoyed not only by the three of us, but by ward staff who frequently came in and were welcome. Each time my parents brought in another box of slides, I would carefully label them. For this purpose I had my map of Austria and street map of Vienna brought into hospital. My meticulous labelling, complete with map, caused much hilarity, but I didn't mind. In fact it was quite funny. Here was I, facing an operation which at the most optimistic gave a 30% chance of survival, labelling slides so as to remember in the future precisely where they were taken! It was rather like Luther saying: 'If the world were to end tomorrow, I would still plant a tree today.'

I was now in a sub-ward of four beds. One fellow occupant was a little girl of five, suffering from meningitis which had been surgically treated. She was one of the most courageous five year olds I have ever met, but had an almost pathological fear of injections. For most of the day her parents or her grandmother took it in turns to be with her, the first shift beginning soon after breakfast with the arrival of father. I soon discovered that a major problem was getting someone to talk Fiona through her breakfast, otherwise what she ate was negligible. On the first day I was able to get out of bed on my own, I decided to take the matter in hand. Taking my breakfast roll over with me, I tried to persuade her to have a mouthful when I did. When a staff nurse came in to see whether Fiona had touched her breakfast, she found me perched on the bed, the breakfast almost consumed and a hearty conversation in full flood between mouthfuls of cereal! Before long there was no need for pretence, and I was getting requests from Fiona as to when was I coming to help, even after she was moved to a single room.

When the hospital first planned the conversion to the Ganymede system of catering, with the individual tray and multi-menu, I doubt whether they fully realized the extent of the new social phenomenon they were introducing. I had noted in my own patients how important was the choice of any combination of selected dishes. What I had not realized was exactly how much of a stimulus it could be in encouraging a sick person to eat. Even more, for the patients it set up a whole new code of dealing with life and with each other. I had always guessed it might be there; now I had the proof. Every morning there was the shared ritual of handing out and completion of the menu cards for the following day. Patients on diets were told the type of foods they were allowed, and then told to mark anything on the day's menu they liked: the dieticians would work out a balanced menu, as far as possible, using the marked dishes. The sound of the meal trolley clattering noisily along the ward produced an air of excitement among patients aware of their surroundings. Frequently the task of distributing and collecting menus was entrusted to some of the mobile patients. They were able to spend more time on it than the nurses, and it was a very different experience to have a fellow patient take a positive interest in your eating than from someone who is paid to do so. Often the mobile male patients would also help with the deliveries. It was good for the other patients to see people on their feet, managing. It also provided support for the men involved, because they received encouragement and praise from most of the patients to whom they went to deliver a

16

meal. Equally important was the inquest after a meal, the mutual discussion about what sort of a bargain each of the dishes had proved to be.

Being a ward of units, male and female, in which many patients would be acutely or chronically ill, room allocation would frequently cause the Sisters difficulties. After the Sisters discovered that, when mobile, I liked having a room to myself, I was moved more than most. My parents lovingly shuffled their own mealtimes, obeying hospital directions: supporting me seemed naturally and unquestioningly their first priority. They and I had come to know and respect my surgeon from the time of the previous haemorrhage, both the hospitalization and the progressively diminishing out-patient checks, without realizing why. Years at university, and primarily my social work and psycho-dynamic training had taught me the reasons.

He is a very sensitive man who finds it difficult to cope within himself with the knowledge that while operating to save someone's life, there is almost certain to be some loss of movement, memory or sensitivity. Deep down inside there is a corner which blames himself, and therefore does not want to befriend patients before he knows they are going to survive. He knows that by doing so he is going to be hurt, and being hurt, that it is more difficult to be objective. He knows that every time he opens a skull and works inside there is bound to be damage. Can the personality withstand it? In my case, I had survived and he had befriended me. He was going to find it doubly hard now to operate and withstand the aftermath on someone he had known intermittently for seven years. That was why, when I had realized what was happening in the cafeteria, my first thought, warm and almost protective, was for my surgeon. I would have to try to convince him that his previous decision had been correct, by maintaining my momentum until the operation.

Intensely aware of this necessity to maintain my morale, music came to my aid. Music lets you drown without the necessity of explaining in words. When alone and the emotion becomes too large to contain, I sometimes find myself conducting. This habit originates from the enjoyment derived in childhood. Music has always been an integral part of the life

17

of our family, from the time when both my brother and I were extremely young. My parents have influenced each other's taste. Father introduced my mother to Beethoven, Mozart, Wagner and Bruch; my mother heightened my father's awareness of Lehár, Waldteufel and the Strauss family. In our turn, we had introduced our parents to the merits of composers like Vivaldi, Fauré, Britten and Richard Strauss. As we became older, we had developed a diverging interest in folk music and I had learnt to play two minor wind instruments. As children, our parents occasionally took us to the Albert Hall for concerts, Highland Gatherings, or visiting foreign dance groups. We had become fascinated by the role of the conductor, so my father taught us the rudiments of conducting, and before long my brother and I were happily 'conducting' everything from recordings of the Berlin Philharmoniker to my school orchestra!

Knowing what music meant to me, my parents had brought my transistor radio into the hospital, complete with ear-piece, and the *Radio Times*. It was to cause a considerable re-establishment of reality in my daily life. One Friday evening in mid-September I was in my room, ear-piece in, listening to Beethoven's Ninth Symphony being played at the penultimate Promenade Concert. Carried away by the intensity and power of the fourth movement, I had begun conducting. Suddenly the door opened and a staff nurse came in. How long she had been looking through the window in the door, I will never know. Blushing scarlet, I lamely muttered something about Beethoven's Ninth. The supporting spell was broken.

Early the following week I discovered that my parents had been somewhat belligerently approached by one of the Sisters. She had asked whether I had ever been so euphoric and unbalanced before. Icy fear gripped them both. I had been my usual self earlier in the day. Sister explained disparagingly that I had been caught conducting to the radio, and that I laughed outrageously at things which weren't funny. My mother sprang to my defence saying that all humours are individual, perhaps mine was just more developed than most. My father commented almost nonchalantly that if she considered the practice unbalanced, then both he and my brother would come into the same category as we were all afflicted with the same response to musical enjoyment. He finished by asking her whether she never did the same thing herself! This was too much for Sister and perplexed, she retired hastily, saying that she had written into my records that I was a euphoric personality.

My mother was particularly distressed that something so damning and untrue should be written into my medical records from a Sister's disbelief that this was, for me, within normal bounds. Fortunately soon after they happened to meet my social work colleague Elisabeth, who said it was ridiculous, I was always like that! She also said she would have it obliterated from my records, after she had seen the Sister. I was very grateful for this as I knew what serious consequences such comments could have to my employment within the Health Service. However, I knew to what the Sister was referring.

I silently discussed with myself: I had to maintain positive momentum towards the operation and the future. If I was going to have any chance to do my part in the work of surviving, I had to keep my morale high. I felt that I had a responsibility to survive if I could, as so many people were praying for my survival. I also knew that my surgeon would inwardly blame himself if I died. It would have been a simple matter if I had a definite day or week in which the operation would take place, but all I had was just an empty, hopeful void. Every time my surgeon seemed to discuss the operation with me, it was to announce another delay. So at the risk of being labelled a crank, I squeezed laughter from the hundred-and-one everyday amusing little incidents that constitute hospital life, knowing that each time I laughed it was a little more than the incident really deserved, but was building a reserve store of positive stimuli into which I could dip whenever I was feeling low, tired, or was in pain.

Many friends, when they heard of my illness, responded magnificently with letters or bouquets. Others, and some of my patients as well, would arrive downstairs in the hope of seeing me, to be turned away disappointed. When I became conscious of my surroundings, there were two large bouquets from Harry, and also a letter from him with a quotation from Romans 8:

And yet, in spite of all, overwhelming victory is ours through Him who loved us. For I am convinced that there is nothing in death or life, in the realm of spirits or superhuman powers, in the world as it is or the world as it shall be, in the forces of the universe, in heights or depths – nothing in all creation that can separate us from the love of God in Christ Jesus our Lord.

I smiled at Paul's belligerent confidence, and retrieved the letter time and again. I also knew, but it helped to be reminded by someone who was not living through the present time. It was also good to have Harry's confidence in my capacity for survival and his lovely succinct comment about my overworking as 'bending the bow'.

From my father's colleagues at work, many of whom I had known from working amongst them during my summer vacations, the response was spontaneous and devastating: a vast bouquet of dark red roses. The love and thoughtfulness was overwhelming, creating wobbles in the pit of my stomach. Before very long bouquets were pouring in from Scotland, Canada, England, and my room took on the appearance of a florist's shop. Aware that other rooms, and particularly the wards, looked forlorn compared with my joyful greenhouse, I began despatching flowers to any of the rooms that I noticed in passing looked desolate. I felt buoyed along by all the spontaneous, caring response: survival would mean reaching for the skies, but with all the support at least I would not be starting from the ground.

Most of my inquiring patients were quite content to be turned politely away, the exception being one persistent lady with whom I had had a particularly supportive role. She had come to my attention because her husband had terminal cancer. He had been complaining bitterly of problems with his wife who had herself some years before been successfully treated for cancer. I discovered that for years she had been made a scapegoat by her husband and his relations, and that underneath was a woman crying out for help. Seeing and assessing the problem, I had begun working with it, aiming at relieving her and mobilizing her many admirable qualities to help her husband. This haemorrhage had come just when

20

we were getting to grips with the problem. Somehow she had discovered my love of red roses and pink carnations and took it upon herself to see that I was never without, though she had run a gauntlet of suspicion and disapproval every time she left them for me. I knew what she was saying through the flowers, but did not feel strong enough to insist on seeing her.

During this period my room became a gathering point in coffee breaks for the unit paramedical staff whom I knew. They were a lively crowd and I enjoyed hearing the news of the social work department. I was particularly concerned that social work in the Radiotherapy Unit should not be neglected, and was very thankful that my case records were up to date. In most cases it should not be too difficult to pick up from where I had left off. I tried to restrain myself from the temptation of giving advice; social work is a profession of decisions. If I commented any more, it might be mistaken for over-anxiety. The unit's head physiotherapist pressed my surgeon to allow me to attend physio sessions in the department downstairs where the range of equipment was much larger than on the ward. I was enthusiastic simply for the change of view; I had been thinking too much. However I recognized the reasons for the refusal.

The whole situation was so confusing. It seemed I was being told so many things by God which I could only half grasp. I had believed He intended me to be appointed to the post in the hospital, particularly once I started to see results. Was this illness His way of removing a failure? I squirmed inside, churning over recent events, looking for where I had gone wrong. It was not difficult to find negative incidents, but there was the indisputable evidence that perceptive relationships on my unit had been improving since my arrival. During the previous few years I had become less scared of letting God take the initiative, without trying to intervene. It was very difficult: I kept finding that, however hard I tried, I was continually butting in. Too uncertain; too little faith.

As I had managed to relinquish more and more possessive desires, I had found a new freedom. It had been exciting walking straight at a cliff edge a few paces away, and each time I had taken a step, to find more firm ground appearing in front of my feet. But now the edge was right here and I

21

was being asked to step into the void. In fear and trembling, painfully aware of my own weakness, I obeyed – to find solid ground under my feet. Never had solid ground felt so good. Gingerly I tried another step, then another and another, each step building up my confidence and ultimately producing the open, ecstatically grateful acknowledgement that God was in total control. Theoretically, I had nothing to worry about. I did worry, but never about survival. That was God's decision. If it was to be death, I could only hope that, for Christ's sake, I could die well.

I was concerned that I was fast becoming far too settled with life inside the confines of the ward, and ceasing to notice what happened outside. I was relaxing into the safety of hospital routine. It was vital that I kept the spring of my readiness to cope and survive after the operation wound up tight. If I relaxed now the spring would probably slacken too far to give me enough post-operative leverage, when I would most need it. As a measure of defence, I began buying and reading a daily newspaper to keep my mind alert to the outside world.

One evening during the third week of September, my flat-mate Jane was allowed to visit me for the first time. I was delighted, not only to see her cheery smile and to realize how well she had accepted my illness, but also for the deeper reason that the hospital recognized my improvement. Jane had been on holiday with a friend in France at the time of my collapse, so we had much news to exchange. She told me of adventures in Paris, which recaptured scenes from visits made whilst I was still at school. I could visualize places and atmosphere, almost smells, as she spoke, the traffic around the Arc de Triomphe, Montmartre, delighting in the heightened awareness which my dangerous position lent me. Why couldn't one be so aware continually, as an everyday matter? It would make life so much more enjoyable.

One afternoon my surgeon appeared on the ward in theatre gown, cap, leggings and shoes, to check the condition of one critically ill patient. The ward was crowded with visitors and the green shrouded figure looked incongruous amongst the superficial gaiety. After the checks were finished, he came across to speak to my parents and me. He promised that they would arrange the operation in the near future, and retracked over the statistical probabilities: 35% chance of surviving as far as the operation, 20% of surviving the operation and the period immediately following, increasing to 50% once I had survived two or three days. I worked out that the overall probability of my surviving was about 10%. The surgeon warned me that as a result of the operation my right arm and leg might be affected as much as, or possibly more than, in 1967. He also said that I might have a slight hesitation in my speech, but he emphasized that it would be minimal and would soon disappear. I was relieved that, if the worst came, I would be able to go around in a wheelchair. Providing I could still talk and communicate I would still be able to work. The thought of being a permanent cripple in a wheelchair made me turn cold. It would mean total readjustment, viewing everything from half-height, no reaching up, absolutely no dancing, no living on the fourth floor without a lift. I made myself face the possibility squarely and directly. Once I had faced the risks, they retreated to the back of my mind; no point in dwelling on them unnecessarily. One glimmer of consolation I told myself would be learning to drive a wheelchair, preferably an electric one! I also consoled myself that whatever else I lost, my speech would remain.

CHAPTER FOUR

Preparations

One today towards the latter half of September, when my surgeon was apologizing for the need to give me lumbar punctures, I said: 'Well, providing you don't give me another lumbar air!' He looked at me, surprised by the vehemence of the statement. I explained as gently as I could why this had remained the most nightmarish experience of my life.

During my time in hospital after the first haemorrhage, I had been given a lumbar air to check the healing at the site. I had been given an injection which was supposed to remove the pain, but leave me capable of movement. In fact it had done the reverse. I had realized it first when the porters had helped me off the bed and, once vertical, I could not support my own weight. The porters had thought they were walking me across the floor: although they did not realize it, they were actually dragging me. I remember it vividly; my feet turned over and I was powerless to turn them back. They were dragging the upper side of my feet across a ridged stone floor. By this time I had also discovered that the anaesthetic had deprived me of speech.

The doctors had earlier explained that they would remove some cerebral fluid from the lumbar region of my spine and create an air bubble which would then be run up into my brain. Once it was there, I would be lain flat and my head shaken gently and systematically from side to side, while the state of healing at the site was checked. I had been man-oeuvred into the chair, part of the large piece of equipment in which the test was to be done. The doctors had asked me to put my arms over a bar. I had, so I thought, but looking down found that my arms had not moved at all. My arms felt extraordinarily heavy. There was still no movement. I was horrified at the deprivation, and at the reactions of the

24

theatre staff who were shouting at me because of my assumed non-co-operation.

When I had been transferred to a trolley, after the removal of the fluid, they had not attempted to make me move for myself. Every slight movement, every jolt, had been a sudden experience of hell. My head was on fire with pain. The effect was made worse by my enforced dumbness, caused by the strange reaction of the anaesthetic. Suddenly I heard the Sister saying in a distraught voice: 'She's being sick all over the floor!' My only thought was that it was fitting retaliation!

My surgeon was now silent. I felt sorry for him; I was confronting him with an experience which had happened seven years before. Yet I thought he should know my feelings in case he wanted to do another this time, and I refused. I seriously doubted whether I could maintain my momentum and withstand all that pain again. After a short silence, he said that nowadays they were performed under a general anaesthetic. This puzzled me because on the previous occasion I had been told that the consciousness of the patient was an important contributory factor in the success of the procedure. I commented about this. My surgeon explained wryly that during the preceding seven years there had been considerable advances and now the only after-effects were the customary splitting headache and vomiting which follow a normal lumbar puncture. I then said that as I would not be conscious to experience the horrors a second time, I would be willing to have virtually anything which he regarded as necessary.

The following morning, perched casually on my bed, he explained that he had to go to Geneva for one week to fulfil a lecturing commitment, and that he did not want to operate when he would have to be away at the most critical point. I respected his reasons for the delay, but my heart sank. The rubber thread of my volition was every day becoming more and more stretched. Instead of my natural bounce, it was almost all consciously forced to maintain momentum. One day it would break. I knew that I just had to survive that week, and survive it well for the sake of similar cases in future. If I did not, I should be betraying all those people with similar problems who could have coped. The surgeons and doctors were investing so much hope in me that if I failed, I felt it would be a long time before they would risk themselves again. There was no choice.

My surgeon also explained that he was sending my parents home for that week, so I should have to manage without both forms of support. For my parents' sake I had to agree with him. Although for the main part they had remained cheerful, I had watched them both become greyer and more haggard. They needed a break, particularly as they had been warned to come back prepared for an indefinite stay. I was determined to hide the feelings of desperation which their departure was causing within me, to save them from feeling guilty about leaving me. The weight of sitting forcibly on my emotions could not last for long. The lid of my emotional box did not give way, but the sides began to crumble.

Although I had said little my parents knew I was anxious about having my head shaved, so a few days before they left they came into the ward in triumph, brandishing a parcel. It was a wig – and the match was incredible. I was breathtaken and silenced. If my own hair had not been straight from weeks in hospital, or the wig not quite so curly, it would not have been possible to distinguish the one from the other. The other patients in the ward joined in the fun and urged me to put it on. Suddenly I, who am normally outgoing, became embarrassed and shy. 'This isn't like you!' I thought. 'Go on! Their laughter won't hurt you!' It felt strange, fitting my scalp like a cap, but flapping round my face; the strange feel of hair not my own round my neck. Several nurses came in to investigate the commotion and joined in the laughter and amazement about the exactness of the match. Later my surgeon came in, having heard about it on the grapevine, wanting to see for himself. 'How kind of him,' I thought. 'He's got plenty to do before he leaves for Geneva, yet he'll spare time to see a patient try on a wig.'

It was the end of the third week in September. The geese had been flying south for days, and in the mornings the mist had the chill of autumn. With memories of mountains, the migrating geese brought an irrational lump to my throat and the sting of tears behind my eyes. Having loved life, I was mourning my own death. The geese, which have been flying exactly the same route for thousands of years, were a reminder of man's mortality. I was very grateful to Jane, who had invited my parents to move into the flat on their return, which would provide a more spacious base than their little caravan. Father would be able to use our drawing-room as a makeshift office, enabling him to work. We discussed ways in which they could smooth Jane's path before her. Although by nature rather reserved, Jane had responded magnificently. The least we could do was show our appreciation.

The response of the minister of St Giles', the church to which I belong, was as tremendous as it had been seven years previously: a different team of ministers but the same rock solid faith, open caring support and willingness to talk about subjects other people usually avoid. The most frequent contact was the Rev Iain David Hume, a gentle young assistant minister with acute perception and an infectious sense of humour. I could release my anxieties on him, knowing that they would not be misunderstood, and receive in return the boundless support of one who also knows the laughter of the Lord. I suggested my parents attend services at St Giles', relying on God to arrange the service and sermon they needed. My mother has long said that she gets much more from a church when not attending a service, but holding my tongue, I was simply pleased that they were finding such support at St Giles'. They needed it and the little I was capable of giving felt grossly inadequate.

The week they were away passed very quickly and, to my joy, I was allowed normal visiting. One unexpected visitor was a country dancing friend who had a brain tumour which was being treated with radio-therapy. Denise was seeking an informed listener who would not scorn or ridicule her fear. She desperately wanted to know whether she would live, to be reassured. I gently said that I did not know. Then almost as an afterthought I asked her whether she had been given any idea about what her chances of survival were. She gave the figure of 50%. Grinning, I told her about my 20% chance of surviving the operation and tried to radiate confidence. It had the effect I was hoping; Denise stopped carrying the burden alone – there was a companion who had even less hope. Unfortunately, despite the statistics, Denise died and I survived.

Another evening the door of my room was thrown open enthusiastically to reveal my semi-housebound neighbour and her daughter. Mrs Smith carefully deposited her large, uneven weight in my chair and tucked her walking stick out of the way, all the time recounting amusing little snippets of local information. She and her daughter poured out a continual stream of life, laughter and care. Mentally, I stood back and surveyed the scene appreciatively: the open response, the love to someone in need. The Greeks had a word for it: agape. Thank you, Lord, for allowing me the additional level of perception with which to appreciate the intensity of people's caring, much of which they did not even see themselves. I wondered why it was that only when survival was improbable did one develop this additional dimension.

Two or three days before my surgeon was due back from Geneva, I found myself developing a cold. A very ordinary common or garden cold! Knowing how reluctant the medical profession are to give anaesthetics under these conditions, I watched the symptoms like a hawk watching prey. When willpower was blatantly of no avail and the cold was becoming established, I requested medication. In the Consultant's absence, the Ward round was being taken by two Senior Registrars. While they dithered, discussing the fact that they didn't think that anything had been developed which worked on the common cold, I suggested a drug at one time prescribed by my G.P., which had acted swiftly and efficiently. They were so absorbed in their theoretical discussion that I might as well not have been present! Didn't they realize how fine had become the tight-rope on which I was walking? They decided to wait and see how it developed. I could have banged their heads together and began to feel sorry for ever having mentioned it. If God intended me to die now, nothing they could do would keep me alive. Operate now and at least I knew that I could go down with all colours flying. Delay and I might still go down, but a shivering wreck, which would do nobody any good, least of all the survivors. Although I continued my relationships with patients, nurses, auxiliaries and cleaners as though nothing had happened, with doctors and

Sisters, I found myself leading an aggressively pro-operation campaign and becoming generally objectionable.

By the day of my surgeon's return, I was half-dreading the worst. 'What's all this I've been hearing?' He smiled. I knew him well enough now to know that had he been planning another postponement, he would not have responded so warmly. All my anxiety melted like ice in the Gulf Stream. He said that as the cold did not seem all that bad, there was no reason why we should not continue as planned. I had no need to answer: he could see the relief in my face. I could have hugged him.

My parents had telephoned each evening to find out how I was. The staff, encouraged by my enthusiastic response, never failed to tell me when they had phoned. Twice, in slack periods, I was invited to the telephone by Sister to have a brief word with them. The first time I was so surprised that I almost ran down the ward. It was the first time I had been able to achieve anything approaching a run in seven years. As a result of the previous haemorrhage, the muscles in my right leg had gone permanently into spasm. The second haemorrhage relaxed them. Over the seven years, almost without realizing it, I had developed compensatory techniques to make my unbalanced walking appear normal. Now I joyfully unlearnt the techniques acquired so painstakingly. Automatically, my mind had gleeful visions of being able to do highland dances again. I put a heavy clamp on such fantasies. The wheelchair was the more realistic prospect.

My parents travelled north on September 30th. Although they had warned me not to expect them till the following day, because I was mentally travelling with them, estimating their progress and visualising the part of the road they were on, by mid-afternoon I realized that if my estimations were correct, they should arrive in the middle of visiting hour. They had felt quite excited climbing the stairs, hoping to surprise me with their unexpected arrival, but were deflated when, although I kissed them with delight, I did not seem at all surprised. However they were fully compensated by the warm welcome from the staff.

After a journey of four hundred miles, the ninety-seven steps to our fourth floor flat in Georgian Edinburgh seemed

29

like a mountain climb. I lay in my bed mentally making journey after journey with them. I only hoped that my father would have the forethought to take his heavy electric typewriter upstairs at the beginning. As my mother unpacked she thought of all those people praying for me. Surely God would hear all those voices? After all the prayers in 1967 I had recovered to lead a full, active life, perhaps too active. She had noticed over the past few months that I was having an increasing number of headaches, but realized as she put clothes away in my room and came across quite a collection of analgesics that they might have been more often and more severe than she had thought. She felt that I had known it was building up, and had hidden it so as not to worry them. Had this knowledge in some paradoxical way made me go full pelt into everything? Had I felt it coming, as though time was running out, and so kept driving myself to achieve as much as possible first? They challenged me the following day. I had reluctantly to admit that it was true.

On 2nd October I went to help Fiona with her breakfast as usual, and filled the time until her father arrived by reading *Winnie the Pooh* to her. I had been slowly introducing her to the idea that the next day I would not be able to help because I was going to have an operation on my head. Fiona knew all about operations on heads: she tried to explain what would happen and that I should wake up with a big bandage. She also gently said that I would have to have an injection. Only much later did I discover that on the morning after my operation she had tried to come in to give me breakfast in return. Only after very forceful persuasion by the nurses that I was asleep and that waking might hurt me, did she relinquish the idea.

Later that morning Sister asked me whether I wished to sign my own forms, or have my parents sign them. I signed them, wishing to save them unnecessary trauma. I wanted to carry as much self-responsibility as possible. In fact the whole procedure had to be repeated the following morning because they temporarily mislaid the signed forms! They could attempt a mind-bendingly difficult operation and yet lose a simple set of forms in less than 24 hours! What if I had been a nervous, frightened patient, worried about showing my fear?

30

After the visitors had departed that evening, I was given the customary disinfectant bath and dressed in an operating gown. I reappeared on the ward to be greeted by cheers from my three room mates. I responded with enthusiasm and paraded into the room as though I was wearing the latest Paris fashion. It was kind and warm to know that I had their support. A short while later I received a message that an aunt from England was on the telephone, rather upset, and would I go and speak to her. I was allowed to do so, and tried to comfort her not so much by what I said but by the confidence and cheerfulness in my voice. Gradually she calmed down.

I was intensely aware of every passing minute; the sand in my hour glass possibly about to run out. It heightened my awareness of every passing second, every little noise – staff moving quietly in the pantry, clocks ticking, beds creaking as patients turned over, sighing and gentle snoring from the next bed. One of my favourite staff nurses came in to offer me sleeping tablets. I refused them because I did not want to miss anything of what might be my last night alive. I wanted to enjoy it! I snuggled comfortably into the warm sheets, trying to savour the individual sensations and was hopelessly bombarded by sensory input.

Suddenly I saw an intensely vivid image of the side entrance of my parents' house where we used to play as children. I knew that it was shortly after my brother's birth in the summer when I was three; then Andy in his pram. Then towing my satchel behind me to school, walking on the wide grass verge; playing two-ball against the wall when I was seven. STOP! Slow down. It was all happening so quickly. The film ground to a halt. I tried to back-track unsuccessfully. I relaxed, and was relieved to find the film starting up again. Slowly at first and then faster than ever, like a record played at the wrong speed. Whole years flashed past in seconds bearing all their original emotions with the same childish intensity.

On to grammar school, the vastness when I first arrived. My cycling accident when I hit a patch of black ice, badly bruising my face on the kerb and smashing my glasses. As I relived it, the original pain returned. I saw the Music Room, the Choir practising Beethoven's Choral Fantasia and the music master tearing his hair and saying that we were the only choir he knew who naturally sang in quarter-tones. My first year as School Wardrobe Mistress: the play was *The Taming of the Shrew*, fifty costumes. During performances I ran a fourteen-hour school day, from 8.30 in the morning, ironing in the Needlework Room until 10.30 at night when the performance finished. I felt the same exhaustion.

Memories were racing out of control. Oh, please slow down! The plague of crane flies, the freezing winters, the hockey pitch covered with ice. Cold muddy winters with me as first XI goal-keeper. My school career was passing with incredible speed: coffee and knitting in the Prefects' Room; so much and so intense. 'A' levels: the examination hall stinking of peppermint. Each scene I saw in the blinking of an eye, encompassing all the surroundings in detail; the light, the emotions, the smells, the words. The jubilation at my university admission, Freshers' week, my first ball, my illness; second year English, sitting outside the examination hall.

Suddenly the staff nurse appeared again and discovering that I was still awake tried again to persuade me to take sleeping pills. I wanted her to go so that I could continue absorbing the memory film in my brain, but she stayed to argue. Should I succumb for the sake of peace? No, I couldn't. I was learning so much. I had heard that many people had this type of experience just before they died. I had decided years before that sleeping pills were not for me; for other people, yes, but not for me. Assuming that the experience heralded this future, I dreaded appearing before God and Christ to have Them ask why I had broken my own rule! I had enough to answer for already. Thinking it would finally silence the nurse, I challenged her with this information. She did not know how to react and departed confused. Sadly I discovered that the memories had either stopped or reached the present. I wondered what I had missed. Gradually and very peacefully, I drifted into sleep.

CHAPTER FIVE

Surgery

I was woken just after six by a nurse who brought me a cup of milky coffee, the last thing I would be allowed before theatre. I wrapped my hands around the cup and drank thankfully. The intensity of the previous evening's experience had not diminished. It was like looking at life through a microscope. I must write to my parents. Permission was given when the nurse returned. The ward was quiet. 'Dear Mum and Dad'; I desperately wanted to help my parents and surgeon cope with my death: particularly my surgeon. I wanted to let him know that I had gone into the operation with my eyes open, that I admired and totally supported his courage and that I hadn't minded dying. No, I couldn't write that yet. I must start gently. 'Hello! It's 6.30 and I've had a cup of coffee. . . . I feel in fine fettle. . . . My main reason for writing is to let you know how super it's been belonging to the Gibbs/Marr family. I mean our batty little group. . . .' I deliberately used very relaxed slang language, imagining them reading, taut with anxiety or grief:

You know how it is when kids grow up, they have a vague appreciation of their families and it deepens as they grow older. My insight, for what it's worth, started about my 'O' level year. I really feel that I've had a thumping good 26 years' worth, and wouldn't have wanted to change it for any other family I've met in my time. Other families are nice to meet, stay with, converse with. They're different and give you a different perspective in life, but home is where one belongs. That's really why, when one has some grey matter to call one's own, that one puts 'home' under a microscope when one's there, and defends it to the hilt when you leave. Perhaps you didn't know that I do, but

33

it's true. It's super growing up in a loving, concerned environment and if I've 'turned out reasonable' then you score a hefty proportion of the credit because I wouldn't have grown up the way I have without that environment. . . . I think it's also given me a fairly high tolerance level – which is useful with people, but also in situations like this.

Then I went on to domestic matters, making provision for my possessions. I also reminded them to apply for the government death grant. During these instructions, my surgeon's name sounded repeatedly in my head.

I wanted to charge my parents with the responsibility of helping him. He would automatically, if subconsciously, blame himself: yet to charge them with an added responsibility at such a time would be cruel. I should have to rely on their warmth and humanity. Instead I wrote:

'Now I can express my confidence in Mr Edward and say that I look forward to seeing you when I surface. With all my love, Kristine.' The conclusion was inadequate but would have to do. I sealed the envelope, lay down and went back to sleep.

The day was in full swing when I woke again; no breakfast this morning: I turned over and tried to block out the sound of the other three patients enjoying their bacon and eggs. Eventually I was given my second pre-operation bath and returned to my bed to await the summons to theatre. I watched the clock creep closer to the scheduled starting time of 9.30. The Senior House Officer came in to tell me that the Professor had started a short, unscheduled operation in the adjacent theatre and was using equipment which was essential for mine. I expressed what I thought of the Professor for blocking 'my' theatre in no uncertain terms! The doctor, bewildered by criticism of his Professor, beat a hasty retreat. I was mainly worried about getting down to theatre before lunch because I knew about that time I would start to feel sick from hunger. If I was sick how could I be sure that they would still operate?

The theatre porters collected me about eleven thirty. My first thoughts were of relief that I shouldn't have to sit through lunch. It seemed from my horizontal position that everybody who was mobile came out to see me off. From my bed I waved to the attendant crowds. Sister appeared to wish me luck; I looked up at her eyes; we both knew what I was facing. I left the ward surrounded by natural confidence and sincere good wishes. What a send-off! Even then I was able to appreciate professionally what they were doing.

In the theatre anteroom I was transferred from my bed to a theatre trolley. An anaesthetist came through the further door which led into the theatre. I had always been curious about this celebrated round theatre, with its ceiling of lights. Plucking up courage I asked if the anaesthetic could be arranged so that I might see the theatre before I became unconscious. However it was not possible as my surgeon had kindly stipulated that I was to be shaved under anaesthetic, to save me the trauma of watching the transformation from shoulder length hair to utterly bald. Seconds later I was unconscious.

For my parents it was a strange automatic day. My mother supposed that they had breakfast, but neither of them could remember. They had not had a telephone call by half-past nine, starting time in the theatre, so assumed everything was running according to plan. Before she left for work, Jane had asked to be phoned as soon as anything was known. Mrs Smith met them on the landing with comfort and hope.

Automatically they went to St Giles' as the most obvious place, walking quietly round, absorbing the atmosphere. Eventually they reached my mother's usual sanctuary, the Chapel of Youth. I had spent eleven years in the Guide movement, and my mother had watched progression through Brownies and Guides until I had both arms laden with badges and my Queen's badge. As they went in she noticed a Bible open on the table and went to it. Glancing down her eyes fell on a verse which read: 'And the damsel arose and walked away.' (Mark 5:43).

Stunned and shaken she stood and read it again, wondering whether it could be a message. She went to tell my father and they sat together in the little Chapel, quietly waiting, the clock striking the passing hours. At midday, without realizing they were there, the young minister who was my regular

35

visitor came in to take the lunchtime service. He included a prayer for me. After the service my father came out from where they had been hidden, and thanked him.

My surgeon had told them that he hoped to be able to use a freeze probe to perform the operation. This is a device that is put into the head and by liquid nitrogen will freeze the affected area, thus causing it to shrink and seal. When it can be used it causes much less incidental damage to the patient, being comparatively localized in area rather than a full opening of the skull. It could cause some impairment of sensation, according to the area in the brain in which it is used. The probe was checked before the operation began, yet when my surgeon came to use it, it would not work. It was tried again and again. Everything that could possibly have gone wrong with it was checked and found to be in good order. Why wouldn't it work? It was then decided that the full operation would have to be done.

First my naked scalp was marked out like a chart over the area in the middle of my brain where, according to the angiograms and symptoms, the seat of the problem lay. The cutting line was marked, from just in front of my left ear, up to the middle of the cranium and almost straight down the back of my head to the bottom of my skull. At regular intervals holes were made in my skull, five of them, to allow the surgeon to saw in between. A further hole was made in the middle of the bone for the hook to lever the skull-flap back into position for the operation.

Once inside, the work of cutting, moving aside and clipping back began. Cutting, moving away and clipping back over and over, down and down, the surgeon working through a microscope. Eventually they arrived: the haemorrhage was subarachnoid, right in the middle of my brain. My surgeon removed by suction some of the blood to expose part of the problem area. It was the same area that had haemorrhaged in 1967, but because the old blood was blocking the path, it had leaked mainly in the other direction. The team were surprised by the size of the haemorrhage at site; angiograms had shown it as much smaller.

As my surgeon worked, creating by-passes for capillaries and individual nerve bundles, to try to save as much of my

36

movement as possible, deeper and deeper, he began to realize how fortuitous was the breakdown of the probe. It had forced them manually to work much deeper than they normally would have done. In doing so they discovered a length of capillary which was only one cell thick. It was transparent and could have burst at any moment. If the probe had been functioning, not necessitating the extra work, they would have missed that length of vessel completely. They would have finished the operation, thinking that they had completely sealed the area, and within a few months I would have had another haemorrhage so vast that there would have been no chance of saving me. The surgeon looked on in stunned silence. Before the operation my surgeon had said to me that my speech might be marginally affected, but the extra work had ploughed right through the speech area. He finished the coagulation and delicate manipulation of the tiny fragile blood vessels and removed blood from both haemorrhages by suction.

Now came the task of putting everything back, the brain, the meninges; unclipping the skull flap, replacing and sealing it. Finally there was the task of replacing the scalp and stitching me up. The operation was over. It had taken eight hours, five hours of which were absorbed with rechannelling. My brain had been badly bruised with the necessary handling. Only time would tell how badly my speech had been affected. Normally the dominant side of a person's brain, which governs speech, is the opposite side from which they write – all except 1% of left-handed people who also have left-dominant hemispheres. I am one of the 1%, and the operation had been from my left side. The only thing to do was wait. At the end of the operation my surgeon tried to find out what was wrong with the probe. He turned it on. It worked perfectly! It was nearly eight o'clock and the entire team were exhausted.

My parents had called at the ward at five o'clock and had learnt from Sister of the delay and that I was still in theatre. She said that during the day the nursing staff had said prayers for me and that they were all awaiting my return. Sister had said they were welcome to stay, or go back to the flat and she would phone when there was news. They felt that their presence was an irrelevant obstruction on the ward, so they returned to the flat. Jane was home from work by the time they arrived and Mrs Smith, who had heard their laboured progress upstairs, came to hear the news.

My father telephoned the ward at half-past seven; I still was not back. Sister had telephoned down to the theatre and quoted the message she was given:

'We are closing Kristine now.'

At half past eight the flat phone rang. It was my surgeon. He told my father that he had just come up to the ward to let them know the results. He had been working for eight hours on me and I had come through well. I had opened my eyes and recognized him, and he felt greatly relieved with the results. My leg would be good but my arm would be weak. He would see my parents in the morning to explain more fully. My father thanked him for all his work, patience and care, and for taking the trouble after all those hours in theatre to telephone personally. My parents stood in the hall holding hands, praying that having survived the haemorrhage and the operation I might live.

An audible sigh of relief went round the flat. My mother told Mrs Smith who, with tears in her eyes, clasped my mother's hands and requested a daily bulletin. Andy telephoned for news. My mother rang a family friend who had been particularly concerned and anxious. May told my mother that the previous day she and her husband had been to Aylesford Priory in Kent. The Prior had invited guests to write down petitions which the community would include in their devotions for the following day. They wrote my name. I learnt later that other friends had made a similar petition at Aylesford on the same day.

My head, down to my eyebrows, was swathed in bandages. A draining tube protruded from the crown, feeding into a bottle fixed to the headrail. A drip was suspended at the other end of the bed, fixed into my foot. I had to have complete nursing checks every half hour: temperature, blood pressure, respiration, pupil dilation, stimulation reactions. When my parents came in the following morning they watched a half-hourly check. The nurse gently opened one eyelid, shining her torch close to my eye, and noted the reaction; then the other eye. She asked me to move my legs. Sleepily I moved the left one, but the right one only moved after she had pinched and scratched it. The nurse then asked me to open my mouth. I managed to part my lips a fraction. 'That's fine,' she said, 'Now poke out your tongue.' My parents just saw the tip. 'That's wonderful!' The jubilant nurse marked her observations on my chart.

My parents had found my letter, and somewhere quiet to read it. It had the desired effect. Their official appointment with my surgeon was not until later, but as they went away they met him in the entrance hall.

'We may as well talk now; it's quiet here.' He said that the fault had been worse than they had ever expected. It was central as the plates had shown, but they had never shown how large it was. The plates from 1967 had been compared with the recent ones and it was as if in both cases they had only seen half. The two sets of plates had to be seen together to estimate the full size of the haemorrhage. My surgeon said:

'It was enormous – well, I don't suppose you would think so.'

'About the size of a walnut?' suggested my mother.

'That was just about the size of it,' he replied.

If he had simply removed it I would have been left greatly impaired. He went on: 'I could not have done this. We spent hours channelling minor blood vessels into larger ones to re-route the blood flow. For that reason it will be some time before some parts start to work again. Her leg will be fine,' he said, looking at my mother, 'but she will always have a weak arm. We had to go right through the arm and speech area.' Then he carefully explained about my left-dominant hemisphere. Most left-handed people have their cerebral speech area on the right, but I was one of the rare left-handed people whose brain also had explicit left-dominance. He told them how he had spent more hours removing the old and recent blood from both haemorrhages by suction. This movement and handling of my brain had caused significant bruising. Nothing can hurry a bruise healing: it must take its time. My parents were emotionally overwhelmed by all the information. My father thanked him for all his care and long hours of patient work. His reply was curt and blunt, 'You don't get social workers of that calibre very often.'

At lunchtime my parents returned to the ward to ask Sister whether perhaps they could feed me a drink, but she explained that I could not take anything by mouth. The drip in my foot served a double purpose: it provided essential nutriment and by its physical structure flowed freely through my veins, preventing clots forming in my blood. As she gave them permission to visit me, Sister added that if I was awake, they must not expect any verbal response. 'It will be some time before she does speak.' They looked at the sleeping figure and came away wondering what she meant. 'Some time' was an extremely vague statement, allowing enormous variations in interpretation.

I surfaced to consciousness for a few moments that evening, just long enough to register that my parents were there and that it was dark. I had no idea how long they had been standing there. To indicate my recognition and appreciation, I gripped their hands with my left one, at this stage not conscious enough to realize that this action was no longer feasible with the other hand. It was the first in a long line of progress achieved by sheer will-power. They bent over and kissed me, I tried to respond, but failed; I tried to speak, but nothing came. My head and thorax felt leaden with indistinguishable pain. I had no sensation of my legs and feet at all. Surely this must be fantasy. It was too horrific to be real. One thing was clear. I had survived the operation.

The second time I awoke it was daylight, and the sun was shining. So my survival was real. I listened to the noises of life in the ward outside. They were comforting, establishing the reality of my existence. Movement was impossible. It was as though vast weights were pinning me, trapped, to the bed. Before the operation I had decided that if God had planned survival, I would do my best to achieve it, and that from the time I regained consciousness I would fight for life. But now I was simply too exhausted, so I requested a three day moratorium. I would allow myself to float, to drift for three days, and if I was alive at the end of it, I would accept the gauntlet and get on with it, no matter what the cost. I kept my bargain, although on what I presumed was the third day, I did not feel any better, stronger, or more ready to start a battle which I well knew would not be one isolated fight but a long cam-

40

paign. At the time it seemed quite a conscious decision, although I doubt whether now anyone knows the real truth. I gritted my teeth and put my hand to the plough.

CHAPTER SIX

Encounter with Christ

For the first couple of days after the operation, I did not realize that when I spoke, I was only thinking. Being so exhausted, so drugged and generally disorientated, I did not realize that other people could not hear my requests. It was on the third day, because of the lack of response, that I realized I could not be heard. Because I had always been a talkative person, the realization utterly appalled me. More than that, my voice was the main tool of my work. Whoever heard of a social worker who could not talk? For the next few days I kept expecting to make a dramatic improvement. I did not expect perfection because of my surgeon's warning of 'slight hesitation', but I had certainly not expected to have complete silence forced upon me.

Slowly I developed a system of signals. At first it was merely a slight flapping up and down with my left hand. Some time later I managed to nod my head – not shake, just nod. The staff had realized by this time that my intelligence had not been affected. They and my parents, having checked that my input system was functioning normally, suggested a more adventurous system of signals. Much later it became possible to communicate in sign language, such sentences as: 'Please may I have a bed-pan?' or 'I should like the steak and kidney pie at lunchtime.' The only problem was that with so many nurses necessarily operating the system, the signals would sometimes be reversed without warning. The most difficult time was the period in which I could only nod. Nodding in Europe usually means assent. In my code language, one nod meant 'No', two or more meant 'Yes'. The code was greatly aided when I learned to shake my head: even then I would frequently say 'No' to something like semolina pudding which I can't stand, only to find semolina arriving. As yet I had no choice as all my food was chosen by dieticians.

Another problem at this time was my bladder, retention capabilities being poor. Thus unless there were suitably equipped staff immediately available to see my signals, disaster was inevitable. This distressed me greatly, not only the actual occurrence and the wet sheets, but also the insinuations of retreat into childhood. Closely bound up with not speaking except internally, this became the most dreaded aspect of my illness. I disliked it so intensely that as soon as I had enough strength, I would haul myself up in bed to draw attention to my plight, and hope that a bedpan would arrive in time. When my attempts at forewarning had failed, the staff would be able to diagnose the problem from the dismal expression of defeated misery on my face.

One morning my surgeon came in to see me while I was awake. 'Ah, awake this time, sleepy head.' He squeezed my left hand. I tried to smile, the corners of my mouth flickering a little but stubbornly refusing anything more. My head was full of things I wanted to say. I opened my mouth and strained but nothing came. 'Still not talking to us?' I tried again, still nothing came. My soul screwed up inside and cried. He looked at my parents. 'It's there, but it just won't come. Will it?' He went away, leaving me trying not to let my parents see how low my spirits were. The draining tube had been removed from my head and I now had a smaller bandage. The drip had been transferred from my foot to my left arm. It was splinted in position. Feeling that I had let my parents carry too much of my internal depression, I waved them out, splint, tubes and all. As they passed the windows between my room and the corridor, I saw their eyes light up. I could hear the greeting of the plump wee domestic whose work this ward was. 'She's in grand spirits today. She's getting on fine.' Good old Mrs Macvarish. It had worked; but fortunately God had seen the anguished cry inside.

Eating was yet another problem. Time and again I wished that I could give it up entirely. At this stage I had to be fed by nurses. It took much patience and perseverance on both our parts. My mouth was still badly affected, and I could open it very little. Once the food was inside, chewing was

43

difficult and painful as the cheek and jaw muscles were mobilized again. I became very thin, at one time weighing less than six stone. The dieticians tried to help with lots of milk puddings and blancmange, desserts which I have avoided since early childhood. I tried my best, but sometimes the physical revulsion was too great. My tongue too was involved in the paralysis, and swallowing had become a near impossibility. Any food or liquid had to spend ages wandering aimlessly around my mouth before I found the control, coordination and energy to swallow it.

As my eating capabilities eventually improved, my parents were allowed to resume the feeding rota. They were delighted to do so. In the morning my father worked on reports from Hawker Siddeley Dynamics Engineering, and then came to the hospital to feed me lunch. Meanwhile my mother, who had once been a secretary, typed out what he had drafted. As his output is extraordinarily high, she had to work like a beaver to finish before he got back. If she had finished, she began to worry about his late return, wondering whether it heralded bad news. As soon as she heard the car, she would pounce on him for news, every day the same question, had I spoken? Every day the same answer, no, not yet. In the afternoon she came in to feed me supper and stay until evening visiting, when my father would join her.

When I had recovered from the initial shock of discovering that I could not talk, I assumed that I could still write. It occurred to me that this was an experience about which the medical profession might be interested to hear. Perhaps I should keep a diary? At any rate it would be a rather long-winded way of communicating my day to day needs, and better than silence and having my requests consistently misinterpreted. If all went well and it was of interest to the general public, perhaps I might later reorganize and publish it. Flushed with enthusiasm, I took up ball-point pen and paper.

'No time like the present!' I thought. My pen was poised, my mind racing with ideas. Try as I would, I could not organize the ideas into logical sentences. I could visualize the words in typescript, and just assumed that I was out of practice. I concentrated harder. I knew exactly what I wanted to say but it simply refused to come. 'I', then blank; repeating the action as a form of stimulus produced no comforting results. 'Try something simpler – single letters.' I tried, with a clear-cut single image in my mind, but still produced an indecipherable scrawl. I seemed to have physically forgotten how to write the letters of the alphabet!

With intense concentration I forced myself to write. C A K E. Slowly and shakily I traced 'cake', and stared disbelievingly at the word. I had wanted to write something profound: what I had written was irrelevant. Great expectation was followed by bitter defeat. Aggressively, I scratched it out. It had exhausted and distressed me too deeply to risk trying it again then. Slowly, after several days practice, I began to create recognizable letters. Those like 'd' and 'b', or 'p' and 'q' frequently came out the wrong way round, as a five-year old might write them. Or I would forget the down stroke to change an 'r' into an 'n', or vice versa. The frustration was incredible.

I became very downhearted and sometimes it was only the intolerable thought of remaining in my present greatly disabled condition that kept me battling onward. The hospital staff tried to encourage me, but I could tell from the hollow ring in their words that it had been much worse than expected. It would be far easier to die. O Master, may I die? The request was desperate. Suddenly I found myself facing the foot of the cross. I clung to it desperately; shocked, tense, my throat closed and dry. The wood was old, bleached by the sun, and very rough. I clung, both arms tightly around the cross, the paralysis non-existent. Yet I knew that my right arm was lying powerless beside me. But what right had I to complain considering what Christ had suffered for me? With a silent, heaving sob I pressed my forehead against the cross, uncaring about the blood or the splinters. Like Peter, I had let Him down.

Suddenly I felt Him at my left-hand side, offering His hand; felt His encompassing strength surround me. Bewildered, I put my hand into His, immediately feeling vast strength surging, pumping up my arm. It was like a powerful electric current, stronger than anything which I had felt before, yet which did not hurt. Flooded with inner light, overwhelmed with relief and blinded by tears, I swung into Him. Nothing else would matter now. His chest wall was strong and firm. 'Rabbuni': although I had never used it before, I found myself spontaneously repeating the response of Mary Magdalene in the garden on Easter morning. I had no need to explain the depths of my misery; He knew. Strength flooded through me, all my fear and trembling gone. The sensation faded. I found myself burying my face in my pillow, but the strength I had been given remained. Sometimes later, when particularly low, or in difficulties, I would simply raise my hand and cry, 'Lord', and He would come giving peace, a quiet mind and indescribable strength.

A new student in her final year appeared on the ward. Her face always radiated happiness; she shone love. Nurses gathered round her as moths around a light. Something deep within me automatically recognized the origin of that light. The love of Christ shone through her face. She was a round, motherly, Irish nun. Why couldn't she have appeared on the ward before my operation, when I could still talk? I could have asked her so many questions. Whether anyone had told her of my commitment, or whether she had noticed the New Testament on my locker, or distinguished something from my eyes which lit a spark of recognition deep within her, I do not know, but suddenly while making my bed one day she began to talk about her Order and herself. She looked at me to see whether her intuition had been correct. Our eyes spoke, yes, don't stop.

Over the next few weeks we came to know each other quite well. I hid nothing from her, not even the pain which I so carefully disguised from other people. She had entered the convent almost straight from school, but over the past ten years there had been many changes, and from being almost contemplative it had become a missionary Order. 'No', she hadn't been given a choice about nursing, and 'Yes', she liked it, answering a question which had not been asked. There was no need to ask, it was so apparent, and such a joy to watch her work. 'No', she did not know where she would be sent after she qualified; almost certainly abroad, but it did not matter. Basically one place was very much like another. Suddenly her time on the unit was finished and she was gone.

She was one of the very few people who have the strength to give and not count the cost. I praised God for her and marvelled; always the right people, in the right place, at the right time.

Days became a week. After ten days I was moved one room down the ward. This meant that relatively I was progressing, I nurtured this tender plant like some rare tropical flower. I must remain positive. Every time I tried to say something which I had repeatedly rehearsed in my mind, I ended up, mouth silently opening and closing, looking like the proverbial fish out of water. Every failure lowered my fighting resistance. In defiance I put a metaphorical plug in the bottom of the bath of my determination and kept on doggedly trying. I practised simple phrases in my mind, over and over, in the hope of being able to produce them at suitable times and have a devastating effect on doctors and staff.

Most of all I practised a welcome to my surgeon. 'Good morning, Mr Edward.' Seven syllables; I knew that it would be flying my colours extraordinarily high, yet if I could succeed it would give us both enormous encouragement. So I struggled on, practising under my breath, gradually hearing the indecipherable mass become intelligible. My colleague, Elisabeth, was a great support during these days. She came in and visited me briefly during every working day. After a couple of days of practice I was ready to risk a greeting. On whom better to try than Elisabeth? It came out reasonably intelligibly! The word flashed round, and soon I had an expectant gathering of nurses round my bed. I knew that the hovering figures wanted a repeat performance, but hard as I tried, not another word came.

Later that morning, perhaps in the rush of enthusiasm, the doctors decided to get me out of bed to sit in a chair. My physiotherapist had been complaining about the inadequacy of treating me lying down. A student nurse had been assigned the task of getting me into a chair. We succeeded but I was terribly unbalanced and weak. The nurse decided to tie me in, and turned round for cord. I felt myself toppling forward and, unable to stop myself falling, tried to call. Nothing came. Other patients had seen the beginning of my descent and called a warning to the nurse who turned round, but by that time I was so near the floor there was nothing she could do. In that frozen second, I saw the panic on her face and felt her stomach turn over. The crack as my head hit the floor could be heard round the room. Fortunately by this time I was so resigned to disasters that I was relaxed on impact. A very frightened student nurse bent over me: I tried to apologize with my eyes, hoping that this experience would not put her off nursing.

I was speedily returned to bed with an appalling headache fast developing. After being given analgesics all I wanted to do was rest. The doctors had other ideas; in their anxiety they did repeated sensory checks, frustrating me to the point of anger. There was a continual stream of them for the rest of the day, shining ophthalmoscopes into my eyes, pinching and scratching my feet and asking inane questions to which I could only give internal answers. When my father arrived to feed me lunch, I could only manage a couple of spoonsful of soup. I could see his distress, although I could only tell him by thought process that they were all needlessly panicking. In my exhausted, drugged and pain-ridden state, I quite bluntly and fatalistically faced the possibilities unmoved. I was untroubled whether I died or survived; what did scare me was the thought of half-surviving.

When my father returned to the flat, he seemed to my mother strange, confused, a little lost. He told her the good news first, that I had said 'Good morning' to someone, just like that. She knew there was trouble coming. He explained about my fall and the checks. She stood reliving the events, and saw my fall through the nurse's eyes. As she captured it, her stomach somersaulted. 'Poor little nurse.' Both of them came to the hospital that afternoon, and met my surgeon as they arrived. 'I hear Kristine spoke today,' he said. 'When they told me – well – it made my day.' He went on to say that they were not to worry about the fall. It had been nasty, but he had checked and I was all right. They both expressed concern for the nurse, and said they would mention it to Sister as they did not want the nurse to feel as though the incident hung over her like a black cloud. My surgeon was pleased and said he would also mention it and then asked whether the speech had occurred before or after the fall.

When he heard it had occurred before, he was thoughtful and said that they would all have to be patient.

CHAPTER SEVEN

Pain

The following morning Sister and a staff nurse were standing at the end of my bed discussing the fact that they both thought my bowels needed a little encouragement. Being prone for weeks they had become erratic. It was becoming plain that I would be presented with a large dose of Sennakot or Syrup of Figs. I disapproved of the laxative, but even more of a practice unacceptable in social work, discussing a person in their presence without including them in the conversation. My blood pressure rose as the discussion continued, and finally exploded. I yelled 'NO!', in my head. But it was not only in my head; the sound echoed round the room. Automatically I looked round to see who my defender had been, at the same time knowing that I had been the speaker. A slight hesitation crossed Sister Anderson's face, then a broad delighted smile. She had heard me speak! The threatened laxative was forgotten. I knew that I was on iron pills and that when my body had had enough, it would simply reject the excess.

The half-bandage was removed and replaced by a stockinette cap. The bandages had been redressed daily by a staff nurse in the dressing station, but the stockinette cap could be redressed in the ward and other nursing staff became involved. One SEN began persistently accusing me of scratching my wound. I tried not to, although sometimes it itched almost unbearably, because I knew that if I succumbed to the temptation my progress would be delayed. Only I knew with what battles I kept my left hand battened to the sheets. I struggled to reply to her accusations, trying to tell her, mainly in gestures, that I didn't think I did, certainly not consciously.

A couple of days later she was beside my bed as my consultant's ward round was passing. As usual, they stopped at the end of my bed. Suddenly she said that I was scratching my wound. I was prepared for a nurse to misunderstand or misinterpret what I said if she chose, but it was quite another thing to have my surgeon given such damning and potentially incorrect information. I saw red! Again I bellowed 'NO!', this time with somewhat better volume control. My surgeon came down between the beds. It was now or never; I screwed up every ounce of energy, and greeted him verbally. In my anxiety the 'Good morning' was lost, but his name came over clearly. His pleasure showed in his face; I smiled, much encouraged.

A fortnight after the operation and several days after the fall, the results of checks on the retina for undue pressure became so disconcerting that my surgeon decided to start administering lumbar punctures. I could diagnose when one was needed because the pain behind my eyes became like twisted steel rope. I had fifteen lumbar punctures during my hospitalization: three before the operation, and twelve afterwards. I remember the latter thirteen. The doctors had to do so many in such a small space that they had to move one vertebral space up my spinal column. The punctures had become so painful that I found it almost impossible not to move while they were being done. The local anaesthetic no longer seemed to contain the pain of the insertion of the needle. This only made it worse, for the doctor's awareness of how much pain he was causing distracted his attention and his aim. In such a delicate procedure, if the spinal cavity is missed, there is no alternative but to go back to the beginning and start again. From retina pressure checks, it averaged that I needed two punctures every three days, which eventually, as more and more was demanded of the same small patch of skin, did not allow enough time for the previous puncture scar to heal.

It was at this stage that the pain graph progressed geometrically. When the doctor had done a retina pressure check, I would be told whether or not I would need a puncture that day, and if so, when it was likely to happen. For about the last five I took to cheating. During the general pill round before the appointed time, I would ask for analgesics. I had

51

discovered that the tablets significantly reduced the pain of the actual puncture, thus reducing the probability of involuntary movement. They would also be in action for the period immediately afterwards. I am sure that the nursing staff assumed that I already had the headache for which the pills were intended. My speech was so limited that it took all my resources to say 'Paracetamol', without saying that they were an advance insurance policy.

At first the doctors were able to extract two phials of cerebral fluid with relative ease, but as it became increasingly difficult, it reduced to one. After the occasion when, during a puncture, a staff nurse happened to come round to the side I was facing and found tears of pain streaming down my face, they took to stationing the staff nurse in front of me. I tried not to cry out because I knew that they were supposed to remove two phials of cerebral fluid but sometimes, particularly when I didn't feel I could cry tears because of being continually watched by a nurse, an odd stifled cry would escape.

The trouble was that the body is supposed to be capable of replacing two complete phials of cerebral fluid every day. At first mine obliged, but as demand continued without respite, it did so ever more slowly and with increasing pain. In the beginning, once the machine had warmed up and was running at maximum capacity, it used to take approximately fifteen minutes to fill two complete phials. Then it became half an hour for two phials, then forty minutes; then an hour for a phial and a half, and finally eighty minutes for three-quarters of a phial. The pain worked on a similar ratio. At first the inevitable headache, caused by the creation of a vacuum in narrow pipes from the removal of cerebral fluid, would be slow to start and not too severe. By the last few punctures the doctor would be in a dilemma about the best way of returning me to my room. If he trundled me back along the corridor at normal speed, every slight bump would be agony. If he raced to complete the journey fast, it usually made me sick. Also I used to find the turning of the bed to get through the doors of my room or ward absolutely dreadful, because every ten degrees felt like ninety, so that the orientation of my brain would be spinning before my bed was parked. That was without all the fine adjustments needed to straighten the bed into precisely the position it had left! It was hopeless my attempting to ask the nurses to leave the finer adjustments until my head had subsided.

Again I faced the problems of eating, drinking and using bedpans flat on my back. By now I was becoming so nonchalant and resigned about the post-puncture headaches that I would risk being propped up in bed so that I could enjoy a reasonably sized meal. It was a fine balance between winding me up fast enough for me to eat a reasonable meal to give me much needed strength, and leaving me a minute too long, the pain winning and me vomiting the whole meal. Then one evening, after another fruitless bedpan session, I managed to persuade two nurses to risk a bedpan chair. They were very wary; permission had not been granted by Sister. However, after my stomach and their fears were relieved, it joined the race against time; to get me out of bed, onto the chair and the performance completed before the increase in pain level made me sick.

It was now explained to me that I would need to sit out of bed as much as possible. Apart from being the next stage of recovery, my surgeon was worried about the possibility of a blood clot getting trapped in a vein through inactivity, which could be as devastating as another haemorrhage. The first couple of times I got up with enthusiasm, tolerating the indignity of being tied into my chair. My heart fluttered with excitement. I was extremely thin, my shoulder blades two distinct humps in the back of my dressing gown. Sitting upright for more than a few minutes was a near impossibility, as though I was now too thin to support my own height. I slipped forward in the chair, my arched back and stockinette cap giving me the appearance of a little myopic tortoise. I tolerated the exhaustion and pain for as long as possible and, just before my fighting capacity dissolved entirely, requested bed. It was refused. Soon I was no longer capable of supporting my head; my anxious mother went for Sister and I was hastened back to bed.

On the next day, with a different Sister on duty, I waited longer, trying to discover the time-span which was expected. By the time I was returned to bed, my body was too exhausted to sleep and my determination was at its lowest ebb. This was no good. If I was to progress, and not stagnate or regress, a compromise would have to be found. The following day it was suggested that I got up after lunch instead of before supper. I sat waiting for my mother to arrive, becoming more and more tired. I was not going to give in, certainly not before my mother had arrived. It would give her such a boost to see me sitting when she came in. Afterwards I could retire to bed as the nurse had said, and my mother would never realize how tired I was feeling. She arrived promptly with the trolley. I managed a false half-smile. I was too tired to eat, but forced down a few mouthfuls in order to disguise the real situation. By this time I really was too tired to eat, too tired to chew and too tired to swallow. I tried to explain that I had been told that I could return to bed after the meal.

We asked the first nurse who came into the ward. She went to check and returned to say that I was expected to stay up until after visiting time. Time dragged, my father arrived. I cannot remember what they talked about; I was only conscious of my aching body and my exhausted, befuddled mind. All I wanted to do was sleep. At last visiting hour was finished; I asked the first nurse to appear. Again she went to check, and returned with the same answer, 'Not yet'. Suddenly my exhaustion flared into anger. If the staff were not prepared to accept my intelligent estimation of when enough was enough, they would have to find out the hard way. They should have known I would not ask needlessly. I was fairly close to the foot of my bed. If I untied the knots, I should be able to grab the bed even if I fell. Gingerly I put my feet on the floor, in my mind visions of courts of inquiry if I fell. It was a risk that had to be taken. I reached the bed without mishap. A nurse came in soon afterwards and finding me in bed, asked who had returned me. I just said 'Me', waiting for the storm to break.

The nurse hesitated, uncertain, shifting from one foot to another. She rushed out. The silence hung heavy with threat. I remained defiant, having committed the impossible crime: I had disobeyed instructions. The door flew open and Sister roared into the room. Scrupulously fair, she did not explode until she had confirmed the unlikely story with me. This

Sister had earned my admiration for her perception and caring; it hurt to hear her accusations. Yet I knew that I had earned them. I motioned with my hand for her to allow me to speak. It was lucky that it was she who was on duty, for she would at least grant me a fair hearing. Haltingly, mainly in nouns and verbs, I presented my apologia: 'Want get well, fighting life, badly overtired, disastrous therapy tomorrow, no energy several days give up. Must bed now for tomorrow.' A vast string of words for my present state. Sister said very little after that, but I knew the subject was only beginning.

As I had expected, the following morning my surgeon came in to tackle me about my insurrection. Although I tried, few words came and I was only able to check whether Sister had told him of my defence the previous evening. She had. He tried to get me to promise that I would not do it again. I agreed providing that when I got really exhausted the nurses would let me have a short period lying down, then as soon as I was a little less tired and weepy, I would sit up again.

Later in the morning I was helped into a chair, and had lunch sitting up. It really felt like an achievement. That afternoon I actively fought down the tell-tale sensations, trying to tell myself that they weren't real, that my tiredness wasn't becoming a nagging pain. If only my mother was not there; I would not have to split my concentration and could focus it entirely on staying vertical, coping with the exhaustion and the pain. Every time I tried to concentrate on something else, my head, back or legs would give a sudden stab. Eventually the entire structure crumbled and disintegrated. Streams of tears pouring down reluctant cheeks, I was angry with myself for having exposed my mother to so much of my hopelessness. It would live in her memory, whereas I knew that my good spells outweighed the low, lost ones. Ultimately I knew that I was not fighting this battle alone, but in the arms of the strongest invisible support, so mentally I apologized and kicked myself for my lack of strength.

Sister came in. 'You probably are tired, Kristine, but you are not going back to bed. You know as well as we do that too much bed is not good for you. I don't think those tears are tiredness, they are frustration. You can hear everybody else talk and you cannot, and it's more than you can bear.'

Of course it was frustrating not being able to talk, having my signals frequently misinterpreted and my thoughts wildly misassessed. But if only Sister could have shared the desperately grinding, nagging pain of my lumbar spine from punctures, my throbbing head, the aches and exhaustion of trying to counterbalance my paralysed right arm. I was too exhausted even to try. She turned to my mother: 'If she were a thicky, it wouldn't bother her. It is because she is highly intelligent, she knows things aren't right and it upsets her.' She turned back and spoke to me: 'I know it's dreadful just now, but it will come back. Now dry your tears and have a nice cup of coffee.' Dejected and crying gently, I thought only that that was the way with hospitals. They want things neat and tidy and did not stop to consider that having become grossly overtired, I could no longer control whether I was depressed or not, and was totally unable to stop my tears. So I just sat like a moron until I was allowed back to bed.

I would need strength and energy if I was to become active again. If I went beyond self-retrieval, I would cease to care either for myself or other people. I had looked into the void and knew that I was no exception. Ultimately I was unconcerned about whether I died or survived. It was the quality which concerned me. Surely God would not have expended so much energy getting me to survive the operation, only to fall into an abyss of inactivity afterwards? God knew what He was doing: it was just my too-small faith that kept looking for answers. Recommitting my life to Christ, I shouldered the task of rehabilitation, wielding an unspoken threat over the heads of the staff: 'You can try me, but if you do not allow me bed when I really need it, you know that I'll just have to take myself.'

It had become clear that my right arm would be far from normal by the time of my discharge. Knowing that the washing machine I had in the flat was an antiquated one that had to be hand-filled, my parents began to plan the purchase of an automatic washing machine. My mother set about getting information about various types, and we would talk about them when she sat with me at supper time. I watched her with love, with appreciation and wry humour. Consciously, she was saying: 'Eat your tea, every mouthful helps.' Uncon-

56

sciously she was saying: 'Please survive. See, we are planning a long-term future.' I became worried that they would buy an expensive machine before my survival was absolutely certain, so I extracted a promise from them that they would not take further action until after I was discharged.

At this time my parents were asked to bring clothes into hospital for me. I had begun attending physiotherapy in the department downstairs, and it was awkward, if not indecorous, to have me crawling round the floor in my nightdress. As I looked at the clothes lying on my bed, I wondered how I could ever summon the energy to dress. It needed all the determination I could muster: 'No, I'm not giving in. I'll show them.' For the first few days an occupational therapist was there with ideas and suggestions. When I was stuck, she would help me. The exhaustion of the process left me frustrated. Knowing that positive anger can be beneficial but that negative anger simply eats into a person's soul, and that the longer I delayed, the harder it would be to start, I began slowly raking the muck and rubble into the broad daylight of my conscious mind. That evening, still fully clothed and lying on my bed, I managed a real laugh! Until then, my voice had not managed all the contortions necessary to produce a real, full-blooded laugh. I had spluttered and gurgled, but not laughed. To me the sound was like music.

CHAPTER EIGHT

Oh Lord, Help!

The next achievement was walking. Nan, the department's head physiotherapist managed to contain my enthusiasm in order to develop good technique. I willingly plodded between parallel bars under her analytical gaze. My current aim was to get to the loo walking, rather than in a wheelchair. At this stage an escort was essential. My mother and I developed a method of progress more efficient than the staff holding my arm. I put my good arm round her shoulder, she put her right arm round my waist, and away we went. It reminded me of the days when my brother first outgrew my mother. He would tuck her under his arm, singing from *The Mikado*: 'I've got to take under my wing, tra-la, a most unattractive old thing, tra-la, with a caricature of a face.' I managed enough of the sentence to share the memory and we smiled.

I found people using me as their base-line, the person they used to convince themselves that they were not so badly off as they had at first thought. In the beginning I found it a burden, but after a short while I became accustomed to it. I told myself that if it helped people to stop feeling sorry for themselves, it would be one way I could be of use. Until I was capable of carrying the weight alone, I did the same as everyone else and chose a patient whose condition was worse than mine. Margaret taught me a great deal about silent suffering. She had shocking feeding problems, choking on every spoonful. I was sure that she knew that all the mobile patients evacuated their beds at mealtimes to avoid having to listen to her choking, and watch her vomiting. When I moved into her unit of four I decided that, although recently mobile, I would try to lend her support by remaining during meal-times. Soon I discovered that I cared so much for her that I did not so much notice the noise and mess she made as feel

58

for her distress in losing yet another meal. Her speech was unintelligible and mine non-existent, yet we managed several very basic conversations.

Tom, the resident junior doctor, came on duty at half past eight in the morning. Normally he would still be working at half past ten or eleven at night. When those treating me complained that I was missing important therapy sessions, he took to performing my lumbar punctures at night in the hope that the worst of the headache would be over by the morning, and I could then follow my normal therapy schedule. The nurses had nicknamed him 'the Vampire' because of the frequency of my lumbar punctures. After he had discovered that I sympathized with his frequent fourteen-hour day and eternal exhaustion, when I was in a single room he would creep into my armchair for a few minutes respite from the demands of an extraordinarily busy ward. For the days he was on duty, Tom was on twenty-four hours a day. Like all junior doctors, he was the Health Service skivvy. At that time junior doctors were only entitled to overtime beyond eighty hours, which in a normal job is a full week's work in overtime! The real iniquity of the situation was that for a relatively inexperienced member of the profession an eighty-hour week should have been considered acceptable.

I spent nearly two hours one morning trying to explain to nursing staff that I thought superfluous doses of iron were causing my diarrhoea. I knew my reaction to large doses of iron as I had once taken them for a year when I had anaemia. Now one nurse after another misunderstood my meaning. Eventually I tried to write. My concentration stretched until I felt as though my head would burst. With great effort I managed two letters: IR. I wrote them again and again, hoping that by repetition my hand would repeat what was clear in my head. When it was clear that 'iron' was going to be a dismal failure, I thought of trying to synonym: Ferrous. FE, fe; why couldn't I produce more than two letters when the whole thing was so clear in my head? By now the current nurse had enlisted the help of a passing physiotherapist. Seeing my desperation, they camped down for a siege. DIO, I wrote several times, trying to explain what effect the pills were having. They guessed what I was driving at and thinking that was all, were about to leave. Knowing it would be a long time before a similar opportunity arose, I suddenly found voice and shouted in panic: 'IRON!' My room-mates applauded. Tears of exhaustion streamed down my face. Of such events were my weeks composed. The next morning the iron pill was absent from my daily issue and did not reappear.

From the difficulty in extracting the required amount of fluid during lumbar punctures my surgeon deduced that there must be an obstruction preventing flow. The opthalmoscope persistently registered pressure, but the fluid was not there to withdraw. It was being trapped in the area, which gave incorrect diagnoses. I could tell from the way my surgeon approached that in his estimation he was facing a difficult task. Was he going to tell me that survival was an impossibility? I faced this without fear, and had helpful, comforting phrases in my mind when he began. It was not so drastic after all: he wanted to do a lumbar air to assess what was causing the problem. Having checked that it would be done under general anaesthetic, I agreed quite happily. The aftermath would be the same as a lumbar puncture, and I had had enough of those to know that the pain could be kept to an acceptable level with analgesics. Whatever happened subsequently, the fact that a surgeon had explained and said 'May I?' to a patient instead of 'You'll have to' was a sign of a breakthrough. If future patients were to be offered the sort of involvement I visualised, it was desperately important that I did not fail.

The following morning he was at the foot of my bed with a group of students explaining the need for an exploratory lumbar air. I greatly appreciated the way he automatically widened the circle to include me in their discussion. He showed respect and willingness to listen to each student and carefully maintained the individual integrity of each individual if he demolished a suggestion. Turning directly to me, he said cheerfully that if the lumbar air did not have the required effect they would have to insert a shunt. I went cold with horror.

In 1967 there had been a hydrocephalic baby on the ward with a shunt. It was a metal contraption with a valve, rather like one in a flute or clarinet, fixed to the skull, which was used to release the excess fluid. It stood out about an inch from her head. Although the proportional size would be much smaller, I was horrified at the idea of possibly having to have one. With my sort of profession the risk of infection would be enormous. Hair around the valve would present another risk, which would mean having a permanently bald patch, troubling potential employers and clients, not to mention personal friends. As for being temporary, hadn't the lumbar punctures shown that they only stimulated more fluid?

The shunt would mean another operation: reopening my skull. I mentally visualized having to attempt the long dragging haul again. The next time it would not just be from the beginning, but further back. I faced myself squarely. I simply had not the strength. If they took me back to theatre for surgery, I knew that I would neither have adequate energy nor the determination to start the battle again. If the staff were to retain positive memories of the way in which I had coped, on which to build and share themselves unreservedly with patients, it was important that I did not return to theatre for surgery. Although the lumbar air would be done in theatre, it would not necessitate opening my skull.

If only I could communicate in a non-verbal language. Suddenly I remembered Girl Guide days when I had learned Braille and Deaf-Blind Manual Language. That was the answer! For one morning I spelled out on every hand that came within reach, 'Can you understand this?', in the desperate hope that somebody would reply 'Yes'. Nobody recognized the signs of a consistent code language; people just assumed that I was playing. Friendly staff drew back in horror, thinking that I had become suddenly and dramatically unbalanced. What was far worse, they treated me as such. I was dealt with briefly and at arm's length. The hospital chaplain, who should have known better, quickly withdrew his hand and disappeared swiftly.

I found myself being treated as if I was mad. I did not have enough speech to explain, even if anyone had come near enough that afternoon to give me the opportunity. From the reactions of staff and Sister's obvious assumption that I had become suddenly unbalanced, I became afraid that it would be reported to my surgeon and that he would have me transferred to a psychiatric hospital where, because I could not explain, I would be given inappropriate treatment. Therefore, distressed by the negative response and in desperation lest my surgeon should be informed, I ceased the only language which I could use efficiently.

That afternoon on her way into the ward, my mother met Sister. With sombre look and hollow voice she explained that I had taken a turn for the worse. Panic rose in my mother; I had been all right earlier in the day. Sister explained that I had become irrational and was playing indiscriminately with people's hands. Horrified at first, my mother suddenly remembered that I had been taught a manual language when I was a Guide. She asked what the strange movements were, and then explained what I was really doing. Unfortunately neither she nor my father could speak the language, and in my fear that the wrong story get back to my surgeon, I signalled to them not to mention it. Fifteen months later, I was talking to him at an out-patient clinic about this period. He told me that he had not been informed, but he did know the language! He proceeded to demonstrate. We laughed at the irony of it: the one person whom through fear I had not tried, was the one person who could have understood.

In the previous two months my parents had been through so much trauma that my surgeon explained to me that he wanted them to go home for a rest, and to return in a fortnight's time. The very idea of managing alone over the period of the lumbar air and the inevitable fight about the shunt, made me cold with fear. However I agreed with everything he said, and told him that of course I could manage. 'Somehow', I thought under my breath. 'O Lord, HELP!' I decided not to worry them about the shunt. By the time they returned that fight, and the lumbar air, would be over.

He gave my parents a slightly different version: 'I want you to go home and come back in two weeks' time. We have reached a crucial stage; Kristine's life is no longer in actual danger. If you stay, she'll think it is serious. It will be good for her to think that I feel she can cope on her own.' I appreciated his confidence and fought down the ominous, tell-tale signs bubbling up inside. 'Shunt, shunt,' the voice said. I thrust it down. 'Shunt, shunt'; it was getting nearer the surface. My parents were due to go home the following morning; I could not let them leave with me upset. Suddenly, the dam, burst. Tears rolled silently down my cheeks. I bit my lip. 'Damn', exactly what I was trying to avoid. I tried to explain, opening my mouth like a goldfish, but nothing came. Dejectedly, I pointed to my head. Father took over; had my surgeon been in? 'Ah', and my upraised finger confirmed it.

'What did he have to say?' he asked. I struggled, my lips moving soundlessly. Suddenly came one word, 'Shunt'. My father explained to my mother that this was the term for a valve, and added what my surgeon had told him about it. My lips tightened firmly in disagreement. Suddenly my mother started to cry. I had seen her eyes fill with tears before, but I had never seen her cry. Again I felt guilty that my weakness was causing them pain: they hadn't asked for all this. Before they left, they told my surgeon of my reaction. 'I know', he said, 'and I shall not do it unless I absolutely have to, but we have to do something about that speech.'

Jane was familiar with my progress, having heard daily bulletins from my parents. Now she asked to come into the hospital with my father. At first I was worried about her possible reaction to my silence and weak condition. As she came through the door, my delight was tinged with caution. However, not seeming in the least troubled, she sat and talked, with me answering in nods, shakes and waves. She did not seem troubled in the least, just as though nothing had changed. It was almost too good to be true, and made me feel guilty about having doubted her ability to cope. That evening Iain came in from St Giles' with his wife, who had been asking to meet me. So it was that on my parents' last evening I ended with one of my largest gatherings of visitors.

The following morning, 27th October, I saw my parents off from the end of the ward unsupported. I had the feeling that things would never quite be the same again. Two days later I had the lumbar air. Again, breakfastless, I watched the clock moving slowly round until rescued by the theatre porter. Downstairs in the treatment room he talked, waiting for the arrival of the medical staff. He gently checked whether I knew that I would be given a general anaesthetic. My surgeon had really prepared them well and they were each checking to make sure I knew. I quickly prayed that enough would be discovered to make the shunt unnecessary. The next day my surgeon and Sister came in to tell me of his discoveries. There had been a small flake of dry blood blocking a ventricle and it was that minute speck which had caused all the imbalance, the chronic headaches, the string of lumbar punctures. The fluid level should now slowly balance itself.

However, my surgeon was anxious about a skin bubble at the far left-hand end of the scar, which kept filling with fluid. If it did not improve, it might still be necessary to resort to the shunt, but first with my agreement they would try one last thing. He looked at Sister and asked her quizzically: 'What do you think of old-fashioned remedies?' She nodded and indicated that it was worth a try. He explained that if the swelling did not subside significantly within the next couple of days, it would either be the shunt or a very tight bandage. It would have to be a whole-head bandage, tied so tight that it allowed no swelling outside my skull, forcing the superfluous fluid to redistribute itself round my body. The bandage would only be untied to be changed and retightened. For me there was really no choice.

I tolerated the roaring pain, taking one dose of Paracetamol before the previous one finally wore off. The tablets did not defeat the pain, but they did diminish the violent edge. The only thing that made me tolerate the phenomenal pressure was the thought of the shunt. The very word became anathema and served as a stimulus to endure the tourniquet round my head. On the third day my surgeon unwound the bandage and pronounced it to be working. I gritted my teeth and held on. 'O Lord, I know that I'm getting bogged down. Help me to see realistically.' I had a caring, supportive environment and access to almost unending analgesics. Perhaps the dreaded shunt was all part of God's plan? If this was so, I should just accept it as God's incomprehensible gift. But I still hung back uncertain, somehow feeling that my stance against the shunt was right.

One day I asked my physiotherapist if I could go down to the gymnasium during the afternoon, and to my delight found that because of visiting upstairs, I was able to have her virtually undivided attention. This enabled me to achieve much more. Patiently Nan rubbed ice up and down my arm and across my shoulders to stimulate the nerves. To my involuntary gasp as the raw ice once again hit my warm, bare shoulders, she would say: 'I'm suffering too!' But she had a towel between her hand and the ice. Then she would change tools to a stiff pastry brush and work until the skin was bright pink. Slowly the line at which sensation ended moved further down my arm. I began to distinguish when, blindfolded, my hand was touched with ice or hot water, and to tell the difference between large shapes.

CHAPTER NINE

Ripples Through the Ether

On their return south, my parents were immediately surrounded by friendly inquiries. Their fears were also the community's. Every evening they telephoned to ask after my progress. Iain rang them after he had visited me to say that he had had me saying nursery rhymes, counting numbers and singing simple songs. He was quite excited; my voice sounded the same. My mother could not understand his surprise as, after all, my vocal cords were undamaged. My father's colleagues expressed it in engineering terminology: 'Reception is fine, but just now transmitters are out of action.' At the end of the fortnight, my parents returned for a long weekend. Enthusiastic to share my new-found skills, I tried to speak.

'The', then silence. With the sentence clearly repeated in my head, I tried again. 'The', but the effort of saying the definite article blocked out the remainder of the sentence. I could produce sentences learned by rote from way back in my childhood, like Iain's nursery rhymes and 'Three craws sat upon a wall', but constructing anything original was impossible. The frustration of knowing the words yet being unable to express what was fluent in my mind was incredible. My parents suggested that instead of planning a whole sentence, I should talk in key words. This brought considerable success. So began a series of conversations in which I would say the all-important word and my parents would start plying me with questions that required only 'yes' or 'no' answers.

Exactly the same problem arose with writing; I tried, but co-ordination was broken. I wanted to write several thank-you notes, but the sheer concentration needed to control the pen precluded the production of words, let alone meaningful sentences. After an hour constructing one simple sentence, my exhaustion and frustration were so great that my parents took over. Gradually we constructed acceptable sentences. After half-a-dozen sentences by this painfully slow method, inspiration ran dry. My mother had taken notes, and I copied her words, shape by shape, like a child in kindergarten.

As I began to improve, the restrictions on my movements became more irksome. Sister asked my parents if they could stop me being too adventurous. They did speak to me about not being so venturesome, but I merely shrugged my left shoulder and gave a negative wave. God was in control and had everything planned, so what had I to fear? Even when I did slip, to be caught by a rather frightened father, I was only sorry for upsetting them, not for the fall. The only reason I could find for my attitude was deep down inside me the knowledge that I was safe in God's care. I knew that my activities were so closely bound up with my overall progress that to have restricted one would have halted the other. So I continued, unrepentant.

When my bandage was changed, my mother was fascinated at the fine layer of brown silk across my scalp which I had not yet seen. It took a few moments for the pain to subside to realize that the pressure was no longer there. Then the pain, which was often so great that it stopped me thinking, faltered, hesitated and finally died away. The relief was incredible; it swept over me like a tidal wave. I cried, not with pain but with its cessation. The relief was so great that I could not bear the thought of being immediately returned to the tourniquet, so I requested the toilet. Washing our hands afterwards at the sinks, before a row of mirrors on the wall, I came face to face with my unbandaged self for the first time since the operation. I was immensely relieved with what I saw. My mother could not resist a comment: 'I told you how lovely you looked.' 'Um', was my enigmatic reply. However, the silken fluff across my scalp was exactly the same colour as before, and I smiled at the mirror with pleasure.

I showed my parents my speech therapy notebook. On the first page there were little pictures: 'This is a . . .', house, cup, book, right back to infants' school. But the speech therapist, whom I already knew, was soon able to set me a programme geared to my interests. 'Who is your favourite composer?' No second thoughts about that one: 'Beethoven'.

'What is your favourite instrument?' After a little thought I had written, 'Cello'. 'Who is your favourite exponent of it?' How was I going to write Rostropovitch? After several attempts I managed it.

During that weekend my surgeon came round checking on the progress of his patients. He looked quizzically at me. 'Are you speaking to me tonight?' I smiled and said, 'Hello'. 'Good, and how's that arm?' I looked at it, sending messages, asking, cajoling, pleading, bullying. Eventually shaking my head as an admission of defeat, I looked at him. His reply was to take hold of my hand and lift it straight above my head. 'Now', he said, 'pull on my hand.' I wrenched downwards with all my force. Outwardly nothing moved but I had felt rumbles inside. He smiled, 'That's good. There is power there and it will come back.' He turned to my parents and said, 'The arm and speech will come back together.' I was greatly relieved; it might take a long time but both were achievable.

By now the rota of therapies was well established. Occupational therapy in the morning, physio in the afternoon, speech therapy twice a week. I still had the bandage constricting my head but now another problem was becoming quite serious. Stitch eruptions from the top of my scar, with the swelling, were delaying my transfer to a rehabilitation hospital. Often I had to force myself to become involved in my therapies, sheer stubbornness not allowing defeat. I knew that no matter how bad I felt, I had to keep going. If not, the rot would set in and it would become extremely difficult to begin. People always felt they were the exception to prove the rule. I saw it happening all round me. You have to decide whether you want to recover, and having opted for life, direct all your energies towards survival. I do not mean ignoring the needs of others. On the contrary, they are part of the life for which you are striving, against the living death of stagnation.

Quite often I would find myself sitting next to a patient who had outrun her determination and was drifting slowly downwards. Then I would automatically and subconsciously find myself encouraging her to greater efforts and sharing round the little strength I had. I felt so weak for the task, but

68

providing I trusted God implicitly there was always just enough strength to go round. Slowly I came to a shadowy understanding about the economy of God. A group of patients said: 'Why don't you blame God? He's let you down.' Shocked, I replied: 'But, no, that's the last thing He would do! I might let Him down, never the other way round.' My speech wasn't good enough to express the rest of my thoughts.

God knows the end while we are living the beginning and we have to trust His judgement about what happens and how much He tells us. It is simply that God has a much better opinion of what we can cope with than we have ourselves. If you blame God, who will you hang on to when you feel you can't cope? No one. Although human support is good, at such times it never goes deep enough. However strong your relationships are with other people, they are never profound enough. You may feel self-sufficient now, but in the face of traumatic illness or prolonged hardship, when your strength is absorbed in just stemming the flood of physical deterioration and mental exhaustion, when human relationships cease to be deep enough and your own strength runs dry, on whom will you lean? If you slam the door in God's face, it is you who will suffer the loss, the loneliness and confusion, not God.

One morning in mid-November I was called up early from Occupational Therapy. It was after the date originally planned for my transfer to the rehabilitation hospital, but the stitch abcesses were still acute and at night I was discharging pink blood and pus on to dressings and pillowcases. My surgeon had decided that I should remain at this hospital until the infection was clearer. The Senior Registrar was waiting when I arrived at my little room. He explained that he had come to scrape the infected part in an attempt to clear it. It would not take long. It would hurt a bit but would be so short that it wasn't worth an anaesthetic. I had no reason to doubt his assessment. He began gently scraping the borehole on the crown of my head. As he scraped lower the pain, noise and reverberation inside my head magnified geometrically, nausea mounted. Suddenly he must have touched my skull. Momentarily the room spun, I retched. It was as though he had touched a raw nerve. The doctor stopped; the nurse grabbed a kidney bowl and thrust it into my hand. My vision was still blurred, the nausea acute. After checking that I was alright, the doctor departed. I decided not to allow any more proceedings of that sort without a local anaesthetic.

With time so compartmentalized, days passed quickly. Weekends were only distinguished from the weeks by the absence of therapy staff and more visitors on the ward. I had several devoted visitors including Jane and the ministerial team from St Giles'. Almost before I realized, it was 23rd November and my parents were on their way north again. As I thought back over the last fortnight, I realized that I could show them some improvement to compensate for their eight hundred mile round trip. It would be their last visit to this hospital. Although I had not expressed it, hardly even to myself, my surgeon knew that I would be sorry to leave an environment which I knew so well. He spoke to me about his reasons for the transfer and I agreed completely. His speciality was surgery; theirs was rehabilitation. They had far more extensively equipped rehabilitation departments and in particular I would be able to have much more speech therapy. The hospital had a reputation locally for being a rehabilitation slave-driver. That would suit me. I was only concerned that the new hospital might misassess my drive, my involvement and my intelligence.

My parents had decided that the day when they were allowed to take me out to lunch would be a real landmark. My surgeon gave them permission to take me out not only on the Saturday, but on the Sunday as well. Having looked forward to this day for weeks, I suddenly became frightened, vulnerable. Excitedly they were suggesting lunch at one of Edinburgh's leading restaurants. With my bandage and thoughts of people staring, I panicked. It would not be possible to wear a wig over such a thickness. I touched my head: 'No bandage.' My mother caught the panic in my voice, and subjugated her own long-cherished plans, suggesting instead that we bought steak and had lunch in the flat. I relaxed, knowing that there I would not have eyes boring into me. Wrapped in my father's voluminous raincoat, I went along the corridor to collect instructions and my issue of pills. It was agreed that I should return after supper: eight whole hours!

70

Outside the day was sunny and blustery. The damp chill of November wrapped its fingers around me. I thrilled like a small child to the sensation of wind against my face. I wanted to enjoy all the sensations simultaneously as though time was was very limited and I could not believe in my eventual discharge. Tucked into the front seat of the car, I was asked, 'Where to?' 'Arthur's Seat', I replied. From this large hill there are panoramic views of the city. My father suggested first having a look at the Firth of Forth. It was incredibly beautiful. Small white clouds scurried across a delicate blue sky, dappling the brown hills of Fife. We crossed the city to Arthur's Seat. It was all the same. Life had continued unchanged in this past quarter year. I had missed the city but it had not noticed my absence.

We returned to the flat for lunch. As the car drew up outside I knew that the time of reckoning had arrived. Jane and I shared a fourth floor flat in Georgian Edinburgh. Could I manage the stairs? There were over ninety of them. From years of experience I had discovered that the best way to climb them was steadily, all at once. From fear of being rendered homeless and to prove that I could still live in the flat which had become my home, I managed the stairs without stopping. The last floor felt as though I was climbing a mountain. To my right leg every tread felt vast. At last I arrived and, exhausted, collapsed into my favourite armchair. Home! The sigh of satisfaction was enormous.

It was visiting time when I returned to the ward. As I made my way down the corridor to my room people called out, friendly and relaxed, to ask me how I had enjoyed the day. Their reception made me feel that I really belonged; it would be hard to leave them. The next day my father collected me for lunch in the flat. Jane joined us. Over tea we dawdled, discussing my speech problem in terms of electronics. An image had formed to help me understand the inconsistency in my speech. Looking at my father, I suggested, 'Ripples in the ether?' He agreed, delighted at his non-scientific daughter producing such an apt description.

On the last Monday in November the news came that I would be transferred to the rehabilitation hospital the following morning. When my father telephoned that evening, Sister came to fetch me, but in the excitement all I could manage was, 'Hallo, going tomorrow'. He asked me whether I had finished packing. I struggled, my mouth wandering soundlessly, eventually managing to produce all of a rush, 'Loadsofluggage'. Sister agreed and added her regrets at my departure. She told me that some of the nurses intended to visit me in the new hospital. This confirmed the rather exceptional relationship we had built during these last months. I thanked Sister for all the loving care I had received, and rejoiced that my contact with the staff would not end when I marched, or limped, through their doors in the morning.

CHAPTER TEN

Engage Brain Before Speaking

The various wards of the new hospital were housed independently, each surrounded by lawns and trees. The ambulance drew up outside a long, low building that looked as though it had been built between the wars. With mixed feelings of excitement and apprehension, I climbed down. A male nurse welcomed me and introduced me to some of the other patients.

He showed me where the washroom, offices and lockers were situated, then left me unpacking. Hanging up clothes in my locker, I began to realize some of the import of the information he had rattled off. Transport commuted four times a day between therapy departments and the wards. I would be allowed to walk if I could manage it; the therapy departments were a hundred yards directly across the grass. There were three curtained sinks at which I would be expected to wash myself. I made the mistake of asking how often I would be allowed to bath. I was told it would be altogether impossible so soon, as special assessment and permission were needed. They would see in a few weeks. Meals were eaten in the sun lounge and patients were expected to be punctual.

I returned to my bed and began filling my bedside cupboard. It was a long ward, partitioned into four sections with six-foot screens with curtained windows. My bed was in the first section, nearest the doors. It contained four beds and the nursing station. The lunch trolley arrived and patients began heading for the sun lounge. Most of the other patients were elderly and seemed to 'possess' particular places at the tables. Some of them signalled to me to take a certain chair, which I discovered was where the previous occupant of my bed had sat. The others cautiously looked me over, asked the usual questions: which hospital? what was wrong? when did it happen? how long?, and then ignored me, returning to chat amongst themselves. I made a mental note to make sure that patients admitted in future received a welcome from the patients as well as the staff.

After lunch most of the patients returned to their therapy schedules. Not knowing what to do, I sat on my bed, and surveyed my new surroundings. A nurse came in: didn't I know that chairs were for sitting on and beds for sleeping in? Obediently I climbed down. There was no use this soon trying to explain that the armchair was so low that it would be a major haulage operation to get up, once down. The nurse explained that each patient was examined on admission and that I would need to change and get into bed. I climbed into bed and waited. Unfortunately my reading capacity had been affected; although I could comprehend as before the operation, as yet my capacity to follow print was limited to a few sentences. After that the print would swim and I would find myself reading the sentence three or four times. So I read little apart from my mother's letters, short Bible passages and the Radio Times. That afternoon I came the nearest to being bored since leaving school eight years before. The registrar arrived nearly two hours later, checked my lungs and pulse, asked a few questions which were no doubt on my transfer documents, explained my preliminary therapy schedule and disappeared.

That evening, after the day staff had gone off duty and before the night staff arrived, the ward was quietening down. There was just a faint whisper of voices and the rhythm of even breathing. Why had I worried? Suddenly there was a loud clatter in the corridor and a babble of noise shattering the peace. It sounded as though one of the patients from the other end of the corridor was going through a manic phase. Two night auxiliaries thundered noisily in with the drinks trolley. 'Evening girls.' The last vestige of peace disappeared and every patient on the unit was awake within seconds. Sleep was a pipe-dream while staff clattered around with bedpans. With everybody bedded down for the night, the staff eventually withdrew to the kitchen and the noise subsided. Just as I was dozing off, the auxiliaries returned and seated themselves at the nursing station diagonally across the ward from my bed. They were deep in conversation and made no attempt to lower their voices. Eventually I drifted into sleep, not realizing that this would become my most difficult problem and urgent need in the months to come.

I was awakened the next morning at a quarter to six to find the lights on and the ward preparing for day, as yet two hours away. Five forty-five! Mentally I shrieked in horror and thought of fellow patients in the previous hospital enjoying two more hours. I turned over and tried to block out the noise but was promptly accused of laziness by the SEN in charge overnight, who threatened to pull the bedclothes off me. I heaved myself out of bed and took my towel and flannel bag through to the washroom. It was crowded with women queuing for places at sinks. It was six o'clock in the morning and the whole place was going like a fair. The din made my head rattle.

The lady in front of me turned to talk. I'd arrived yesterday, hadn't I? What was wrong with me? I told her. It was obvious she did not believe me. 'That does not happen to young people.' I didn't bother to argue.

As I dressed I made some rough calculations. Approximately thirty-five patients and five sinks. That meant seven patients to a sink. Allowing five minutes per patient, that meant that the last person could have an extra half-hour in bed. By half past seven the last stragglers were returning from the washroom. Right, tomorrow I would be amongst them. Breakfast with its two-hour anticipation was extraordinarily good. This morning there was a different Sister on duty, a tall, graceful, friendly woman. I watched Sister Hood giving each patient a word of encouragement; she welcomed me to the ward with a smile so sincere that she immediately became a figure of security in an unfamiliar environment.

Just before ten the door was opened by the porter who drove the hospital's internal ambulance. Picking up my speech therapy book and pen, I headed out to it, struggled up the steep steps and sat waiting for the rest of the patients on my ward to join me. Eventually we set off, with me champing at the bit because in my race to progress, every inactive moment during the day was potential progress lost. The Occupational Therapy Department was a series of large rooms with looms at one side, a frame for rug-making, a miniscule printing press, vast reels of cane, several stools in the process of construction and a complete carpentry workshop. A quiet young therapist told me that she would test my performance on various tasks to assess my capabilities and draw up a treatment plan. By the time I was called to speech therapy, I had been taught a method of tying shoe laces with one hand, and the therapist had checked my proficiency with buttons, zips, hooks and eyes, sand-papering, picking up small objects, shape and word/object recognition. Not bad for one morning.

My previous speech therapist had painted such a glowing picture of one of the senior therapists at the rehabilitative hospital that I couldn't believe it was true. Now I discovered it was. Mrs Macfarlane was large, warm and cuddly, the sort of person who automatically spreads confidence and security. I liked her immediately. She assessed my speech. I was almost non-verbal, and when I did manage to speak, nouns and verbs and conjunctions tumbled in disorder onto one another. Mentally she winced at the size of the problem. Would she ever be able to get this girl to talk reasonably again? I gave her my workbook and clung to the glint of optimism in her eyes. I desperately hoped that behind the shaky writing, the spelling mistakes, the omissions, the ellipses and the crossing out, she could see the real me struggling to get out, and that she would be able to devise a programme sufficiently intelligent to be challenging. She told me that we would continue the workbook and that she would set me 'homework' to be done in the ward each evening. We would start with two sessions a day, move on to three, and finally to four sessions a day if I was capable of coping with them.

After lunch it was the turn of physiotherapy, and obtaining directions I walked to the building in which it was held. From the hospital Nan had arranged that I would be treated by the head of the department, and had rubbed her hands gleefully, saying that she would keep me in line. I waited apprehensively for Miss Appin to arrive. She swept through the door exuding energy. She was short and tough, with a grip like a vice and a manner which even before she spoke told you that here was someone who would brook no nonsense. Here was someone used to dominating people, in the interests of their physical rehabilitation. Well, she would find she had taken on more than she bargained for with me. I would work so hard that she would have no opportunity to complain. After all, we were both working towards the same goal.

During that first session we took measure of each other and I discovered that behind the aggressive armour lay a sense of humour and a kind heart. She was so used to having to bully patients into working for their own good that the aggression was automatic. She tested my reaction to pain, moving my arm just beyond its current diminished arc and holding it there. The pain swept down my arm and across my face, making me flush and momentarily go dizzy. My gaze did not budge. I did not move and said nothing. She released my arm without pushing it any further. The contract had been made.

By the beginning of December I had more or less settled in. The following week I would have speech therapy three times a day. Mrs Macfarlane discovered about Harry and that emotional warmth loosed my tongue a little more. She had put the discovery to good use. I looked wryly at my weekend homework: questions about Harry and his family with an instruction to 'write in sentences, please!' How was I going to do that, let alone do justice to the subject? I was already becoming tired from four nights of inadequate sleep. Washing and dressing was long and complicated since here I had no one to give me help. I was missing not being allowed to bath and had taken to having a complete strip-down wash at night, when the washroom was emptier, thus avoiding having to do it in the morning rush.

My pillow cases had not been changed since my arrival. At night I was leaking blood and infected pus on to them and had taken to turning my pillows over so that I was not sleeping on the dirty side; last night had been my last clean side. I explained the situation to a passing auxiliary, expecting understanding and action. Instead I received scorn and abuse. When Sister Hood was on duty again I slowly explained my predicament. She explained that with unfortunate regularity the linen store was empty, and when clean linen did arrive it would only be for a small proportion of the beds.

I became so exhausted with lack of sleep caused by night staff not lowering their voices as they talked late into the night and performing tasks with as much noise as day staff, that I was only just keeping my head above water. At times the temptation to give up the fight as impossible seemed almost overwhelming: to sink quietly into oblivion and die. It was impossible, because I knew when I faced myself that if I succumbed to the temptation the result would not only be living death but also spiritual hell. I had already progressed too far, and it might take years until real death came.

Mrs Macfarlane next asked me to write a descriptive paragraph, which somehow I achieved, though I found it incongruous that she wrote 'Excellent!' at the end of a paragraph which had seven additions, nine blocked out errors and several spelling corrections. Not long after that she asked: 'What do you consider are the attributes that make a successful social worker – and why?' I spent all evening drafting my answer and finally copied out into my workbook: 'I consider the following attributes to be important for the pursuit of social work; a deep concern for other people, dedication in what one sets out to do, stamina and ability, understanding and drive. Also important are the aspects of caring for people, and success must be counted in human terms.' It had taken nearly three hours of hard work, but I was very pleased with it.

The leakage from my wound was by now becoming so bad that it was noticeable within two days of washing my hair. Mrs Macfarlane, who had been a ward Sister before turning to speech therapy, asked one day if she might examine the wound. She was perturbed to see that several days' leakage were encrusted to my scalp, by now covered with half an inch of hair. Obtaining some dressing-packs, at the beginning of my first session each day she would clean my wound. I was very relieved that it was getting professional attention and the basic physical activity helped to draw us closer together. From my appreciation of what she was doing and a desire not to swamp her, I was afraid at first to release my fears onto such a kind and perceptive person. One day after a particularly noisy, sleepless night, the floodgates burst. Mrs

Macfarlane stood the test: from then on I became much more open with her.

I now took myself in hand to identify subjugated anger. Other people rarely benefit from a dose of your anger, nor do you. My main problem was coping with the occasional blatant lack of thought in caring people whom I considered should have known better. I was not angry about the actual illness, but about being cut off in the middle of my work. I have never had the problem of 'Why me?'; simply 'Why now?' I realized that the road to recovery would be hard enough without the added burden of a chip on my shoulder. If God had allowed it, I could trust His reasons. Who was I to argue?

On the 7th December my parents came north again for the weekend. It was important that they did not discover all the difficulties I was having; possibly later, but not yet. As they arrived in the corridor at the entrance to my ward, the bell sounded for the end of visiting time. A nurse stopped them and said that they would not be allowed to see me. My father explained that they had just travelled up from the south of England. The nurse said that this made no difference; rules were rules. My father was quietly fuming. He went to Sister's office, introduced himself and explained the situation. She gave special dispensation for a short visit.

My parents noticed large dark circles under my eyes and an air of tiredness and forlornness. When questioned, I confessed to being unhappy in my new surroundings, the greatest problem being lack of sleep. My mother asked if I had said anything to the chattering night staff. I explained that one night after I heard two strike, when I was feeling particularly exhausted and depressed, I had called out. I had tried to be polite but as the word 'quiet' was beyond my capabilities, I had said, 'Please shut up'. Unfortunately I had lost the tonal contrast in my voice and the intended politeness was smothered. Their reply had been a negative string of abuse. That night I had cried myself to sleep.

Remembering how I had enjoyed my previous days out, my father suggested that they request a pass for the following day. He went to see Sister but returned with a serious face. 'Patients aren't allowed out from here,' he told us. 'The doctor doesn't agree with it unless it is therapeutically beneficial.'

He had told Sister what a lift the days out from the general hospital had given me, and she had said that she would make inquiries. She had explained that this was a working hospital as distinct from a nursing hospital, but saw his point about the effect on my morale if an outing was refused.

By next morning the doctor had not been in, but both Sisters had conferred and had decided to accept joint responsibility. They would allow me out provided I was back by eight that evening. This time I did not have any bandages, and the relief at getting out of the hospital made me accept the invitation to lunch in the family's favourite restaurant without hesitation. I insisted on going to the flat first to change. Once in winter dress and long boots with rearranged wig, I surveyed myself in the mirror. That was better. Now I looked civilized. Jane joined us for lunch and, once I had brazened the stares of other diners and surmounted the embarrassment at having my food cut for me, it was a great success.

Afterwards we did some Christmas shopping until I began to tire, when we returned to the flat. I decided to have a rest on my bed and in the peace and quiet, compared with the noise of the ward, I was asleep in seconds. All too soon it was time for Cinderalla to return. Sister came to inquire about the day and my face was reassurance for her fears. Tomorrow I could go out again. My mother noticed a notepad on my locker and read out what I wrote: 'Clothes, please, St Giles'.' 'You want to go to church?' exclaimed Sister. 'Could you sit through a service?' 'Y-e-s', I replied very definitely, at last managing the so far elusive 'y'.

The relief at being back in St Giles' was too complex to analyse. During eight years in Edinburgh I had had five addresses but only one Church; more than any other place this was home. I relaxed immediately, but it was exceedingly frustrating not to be able to say the creed, or the Lord's Prayer. It took so long to prepare a sentence in my head that I had to plan ahead throughout the preceding words, and then one simple phrase delivered would render me speechless for the next couple of minutes. Hymn singing was just as bad. To sing one line I had to prepare during the preceding lines and the effort expended would silence me. As for any attempt

80

to sing in tune, that was fantasy. After the service the minister greeted me enthusiastically. Iain Hume and others gathered round and to their questions I explained: 'On bail!' To other questions all I could manage was: 'Transmitters not working'.

On the Monday morning my parents appeared before departing south, defying the rule of about visiting out of hours. They said that they would continue to telephone each night. I had guessed that they did but had never been informed. This shocked them because each night they had left the nurse with a message of their continuing support for me. I bluntly told them that the messages were not getting through and suggested that they should not telephone every night because of their telephone bills. If the hospital wanted them, it had their number. But on current performance they could not accept that this was so certain. If they spoke to one of the Sisters, they received an intelligent report, but if another member of the staff answered the telephone, they were treated like little children and warded off with platitudes.

CHAPTER ELEVEN

Christmas

The next morning I went to therapy with a will, striding across the grass. Mrs Macfarlane immediately noticed the difference. It was as though I had had an injection of energy. In Occupational Therapy I was making a teapot stand from ceramic squares on a metal base. If I really worked hard it could be finished this morning. My therapist asked me what I wanted to tackle next. I had taken a great fancy to the little stools with woven basket-work seats on which patients with the use of both hands were working, and I asked to do that. My therapist said it was impossible with one hand. To me this was like red rag to a bull. I bullied her into allowing me to try, and chose a neat wooden base and deep blue and emerald green cords.

I listened carefully; cut a long length of cord, tied a knot around one leg, then twice round one strut and all the way across the stool eight times, keeping the cord very tight. When your length of cord ran out you cut another piece and tied it in. The main thing was to maintain the tension so that the cord did not slacken. Stool-making gave my ingenuity full rein. I tied reef-knots with my teeth and utilized the spasm in my right hand to grip a leg or cross-bar of the stool. The most difficult thing was maintaining tension and by the end of the session my forefinger was rough and red. Periodically, fascinated therapists had come to see how my belligerence was progressing, and had departed surprised. I was turning out a stool of the same standard as people with two active hands.

The battle to maintain my individuality now became quite fierce, particularly with junior and auxiliary staff. To cope with the stress of chronic or traumatic illness around them all day, many retreated behind a front of infallibility. They expected unquestioning compliance and would retaliate in non-physical ways if questioned. My discipline, and that of staff at the general hospital, was self-imposed; here it was superimposed and rigidly enforced from lack of trust. I was very surprised that most of the auxiliary nurses automatically assumed that my lack of speech signified lack of brain power. They would give the most inane answers to my questions and would respond aggressively when I did not automatically believe everything I was told. It became a terrible strain and as it took all my energy to maintain my therapy schedule, increasingly I found myself side-stepping to avoid confrontation.

I would retreat thankfully four times a day to the haven of peace which was my speech therapist's office. Frequently, particularly at the end of the day after six hours' therapy, the relief of knowing that I did not have to fight to maintain my identity would reduce me to tears. There were some periods when every session seemed to end in a flood. I knew that it was causing her stress; I could see it. Yet she knew what I was trying to do and, although she doubted its feasibility, agreed theoretically. I was always trying to go further, to press the rehabilitative function of the hospital more, not only for my own progress, but as a torch-bearer, a pioneer for the other people who would follow me and who would be able to cope with more than I.

The hospital was now preparing for Christmas. I had great difficulty raising any enthusiasm, despite the energy with which the staff were making preparations. Living on four hours' sleep at night was taking its toll. Even the prospect of my parents' presence for a whole week did not produce any excitement, only relief. Each week that passed stripped off another layer of superficiality until there was only that left for which I earnestly cared – God, Christ, my parents, brother, Harry and the intimate fleeting everyday relationships between ordinary people.

Occupational Therapy had turned itself into a Christmas present factory. After the success of my first stool, I had made another in brown and cream for my brother's living room. The constant pulling needed to maintain tension on rough cord had rubbed the joints of my first finger raw. Now my therapist suggested that I try nail-and-thread pictures. I was intrigued by the idea, so she gave me several pattern books. My fascination quickened as I drew out a pattern on paper, taped it to the wood, and then pushed tiny nails into the wood with a nail puncher and taped them home with a hammer. I chose some thread and set to work. The more complex the pattern, the more resentful I became at being taken from positive work for a session of sanding. This involved looking at a blank wall into which a bi-lateral sander and a plank were strapped at an uphill angle. A timer would be set and I would be imprisoned there, sneezing at the paltry pile of dust I produced, while resanding beautifully smooth wood. I hated it; it was so negative. The same plank would sit there week in, week out. They may have been intended as bath boards for elderly people, but we were simply rubbing away good wood.

Jane visited me regularly, organizing my Christmas cards for me and bringing them into hospital. I laboriously wrote them, and fanned the faint spark of enthusiasm which I mustered in spite of my weariness. A great debate was raging about how much time I should be allowed out. At the beginning of Christmas week the debate was still in progress between the supporters of all Christmas Day, those of the afternoon, and those of both afternoons, Christmas and Boxing Day. It reached a head when the ward doctor telephoned my surgeon to gain support for the Christmas afternoon school of thought. My surgeon's response was immediate and devastating: I was to be allowed out of hospital for the whole week that my parents were to be in the flat. I was stunned; this was beyond my wildest dreams. It would mean a whole week of undisturbed nights. I clutched on to my surgeon's implicit statement of confidence with gratitude.

Quietly the spirit of Christmas lit a flame within me. I relaxed into the inestimable strength of God and the excitement of the coming of Christ. One evening a team of change-ringers with handbells came into the ward to give a concert; they were exuberant and rang encore after encore. Even the night staff were quieter as though waiting with baited breath. In speech therapy I stumbled through carols that I have known since childhood. Each day brought greater relief as Christmas crept nearer and I dreamt of hot baths, clean sheets and home-made bread, giving God a wry smile as He again reduced my diminished needs.

On Christmas Eve I received a seemingly vast pile of home-work from Mrs Macfarlane, physiotherapy exercises from Miss Appin and a sufficient store of pills from Sister. I care-fully wrapped my Christmas handwork from Occupational Therapy, labelling each parcel. Before Jane departed to spend Christmas with her parents in England, she had brought one of my cases into the hospital. I packed it. This completed early in the evening, there was nothing to do but await my parents' arrival. I was hoping that they would arrive at the flat in time to unpack and have a short rest before we all set out for St Giles' and the midnight service.

In the middle of the evening my father strode into the ward. My mother was unpacking at the flat. They had been so loaded they did not have room for me in the car and he would tell me the rest outside. The words bore an ominous ring. Once in the car, I questioned him about the bad news. He replied abruptly, 'Andy's here.' Why the dour expression at such good news? Now I would have the opportunity to thank him for his generous, loving response in the summer. Enthusiastically I asked whether my brother's wife had come too. My father sucked in air between the teeth and said quietly: 'Marcia left Andy at the beginning of November.'

Sudden incomprehensible shock: why? My heart went im-mediately out to my poor brother. Why hadn't I been told? My father explained that Andy had forbidden them to tell me because at such a time the shock might have killed me, or made the struggle to survive much harder. During the rest of the way to the flat, my father told me what had happened. It had been a great shock. Although he had quickly resumed his research programme, he was still physically weak and liable to tears, having been very committed to his marriage.

Why, oh why had the haemorrhage removed my speech, now when I really needed it? If I could talk, I could help so much more. As it was, I was limited to the odd word and occasional phrase. My brother needed my speech to interpret, discuss and explain very complex emotions. My parents would try, but in this particular field I had more knowledge than they. I prayed that I might not fail his need too badly and left God in control. When we arrived, he looked up from his chair, fearful and anxious. I went across, sat on his knee and wrapped my left arm round his head.

'Has Dad said?'

'Yes.'

We sat clinging to each other for several minutes, tears streaming down his face, He tried to choke them back.

'No. Go on, cry. It will help. I don't mind.'

In the hall there was a large bouquet of roses from Harry in Austria. I buried my face in them and drank deeply of their heady perfume. Dear Harry, and to arrive on Christmas Eve too: that must have taken some organization. I wondered if he had stipulated the colours, shades ranging from cream, through peach to deep crimson. Eventually I dragged my eyes from the roses to the letter. 'Hello dear Kristine. Your parents informed us about your successful operation and I read happily about your recovering. I can imagine how you feel and thank God for having brought you back to life, though you must have gone through heavy darkness and bitter doubtful times before you saw the light of life again.'

Blood rushed to my face at the accuracy of his perception and in gratitude at his willingness to share openly. I did still get dark, untrusting periods. The letter contained news about his English examination. He described the questions. I could tell he was building up to a crescendo. The results came after the orals; he had passed with Honours! Flapping the letter, I went into the drawing-room and passed the letter for my parents to read. 'No, you read it out,' said Andy. Doubtful, I tried, struggling to get my tongue round the words. 'Go on,' he said relentlessly, 'if you don't try, you won't ever do it. We don't mind waiting.' So I did.

I looked at my watch; it was after ten. 'St Giles'.' Andy was too exhausted, and my mother was deep in Christmas produce in the kitchen, so father and I set out alone. The cathedral was steadily filling with people, some of whom would not see the inside of another church until next Christmas. What was said tonight would be important for them, for everybody. The carols began and the service; the atmosphere was electric. Relinquishing any attempt at key in the volume

86

of that great congregation, I concentrated on words. To my excitement and jubilation I managed one verse of 'Hark, the herald angels sing' without stumbling!

In the morning we two returned to a jubilant St Giles' and a tumultuous greeting from ministers and friends. They would have liked me to stay longer but I had another visit to make before lunch. Before I left the general hospital, the Sisters had asked me to promise that I would visit them on Christmas Day. The ward was bursting with life. It seemed as though everybody was on duty. It felt like a home-coming. The nurses, with tinsel in their caps, were fluttering round an exceedingly well-cushioned Santa Claus complete with costume, sack, beard and hand-bell. Beneath the disguise I recognized the distinctive features of my surgeon. He came across briefly, and I thanked him for my week's freedom.

One day of that week followed another in a relaxed haze, with no strict timetable: a complete antithesis to life in hospital. Other devastating news had arrived in the Christmas mail. As a postscript on his card, a friend had written: 'Sorry to hear of Egon's death'. Surely there must be some mistake? As my parents had corresponded several times with Harry, I questioned them. They confirmed the sad news. Egon had only been fifty-four. In late October he had sustained a haemorrhage in the brainstem for which there had been no hope. Harry had written to my parents asking them to protect me from sudden discovery. He would tell me when he thought that I would be more equipped to cope. I spent two days constructing and writing a suitable letter. At night I stood in the darkened hall with the roses, trying to absorb the unbelievable fact that Egon had been dead for two months.

My parents had again brought the projector with them which provided a more leisurely opportunity to view my slides of Austria. Renewed memories prompted me to talk, my enthusiasm overflowing. However, with speech came frustration. In my difficulties I became extremely sharp and irritable with anyone who tried to hurry my speech. A carelessly interjected word could completely ruin a carefully rehearsed sentence and because my attention had been momentarily diverted, the words would disappear forever into the void. Each phrase was so much effort, each interruption such an anticlimax, that I would become furious when interrupted. I knew that I was being petty and ridiculous, but the harder I tried to stop, the deeper I slid into the mire. It was as though I expected them to understand the frustration which I felt.

Every evening we had a physiotherapy session and each morning my mother bathed and cleaned my scar. During the week there was a very significant improvement in the condition of my wound from regular, careful attention. It was almost clear, and it would now be vital to maintain the improvement. It was with a heavy heart that I faced the family's imminent departure and my return to a barrack-like existence in which I felt trapped. The journey across the city was silent. Turning through the gates, I felt like an escapee returning to prison.

I was given a very friendly welcome by the staff, but when we deposited my luggage on the bed, the reality of my return struck home. The dirty pillowcases which I had left thankfully the week before, had not been changed. They had been on the bed for eighteen days. I did not mind about the sheets: within a few days no doubt I would feel so dirty that it would not matter. About the pillowcases I did mind, as all my mother's careful work would be lost with one night on those. My parents helped me unpack, and with a lump in my throat which refused to be swallowed, came the final hugs and waves. I went to find Sister Hood to ask about changing my pillowcases. She said that today's quota had already been changed. I explained about the improvement in my scar and that I was loathe to reverse it, implying that if they cared to deny my request they would regret the decision. By the evening my sheets and pillowcases had been changed. It was New Year's Eve. Some of the beds were still empty as patients had either been discharged or were on leave. The staff were all in the kitchens, and the ward was almost ominously quiet. The peace was too good to miss, and I was soon fast sleep.

CHAPTER TWELVE

Progress

As New Year's Day is a public holiday, we were allowed to sleep late and were roused about seven. I had achieved eight hours' sleep. The first of January, 1975; what would this year bring? Please God, much progress physically, but that was only half of it. Infinitely more important was following what God wanted, regardless of cost. I had drunk from the fountain of life and had developed an insatiable thirst. I had to relinquish what I thought was right in favour of what He wanted, knowing that although I might not understand His reasoning, every now and then I would receive sudden blinding flashes of insight. I had to learn to stop trying to influence events myself, and to wait for guidance and instructions; I had to learn that if I was unsure, I could wait in prayer. In the past, when faced with a similar situation, I had all too often moved first out of impetuousness or impatience. It would always turn out to be the wrong move. Incredibly, I found myself feeling grateful for the haemorrhage and the added communion which it had brought. Life was going to be far from easy: I had been given the distinct responsibility of defeating the attitude, so often found in hospitals, which regards staff as all-knowing, and patients as thankfully all-accepting.

Therapy schedules started again on Friday, January 3rd. I crossed the grass to Speech Therapy with a spring in my walk. The week, particularly the necessity of talking seriously with my brother, had produced a significant change in my speech. Added to that was a week in a caring environment and eight nights of adequate, undisturbed sleep. Mrs Macfarlane was suitably impressed and produced the hardest piece of homework yet. 'What is your assessment of Britain's fishing grounds?', with attached map, would possibly have defeated me had it not been for my renewed high spirits. As it was I simply rose to the bait and expressed my disapproval of the choice of subject for a woman by writing very formal language. The paragraph began: 'I suggest that the two-hundred-mile limit be extended co-terminously within Europe and that the first twelve miles be the national prerogative. . . .' It continued in like vein. Mrs Macfarlane was delighted and went bounding through to the Occupational Therapy department where for some weeks she had been trying to convince the therapists that I was more intelligent than my vocabulary suggested. At the time I did not know and wondered why they suddenly started treating me with new-found respect.

My next check-up with my surgeon was due on January 6th. I raced through my morning's therapy, laughing at my excitement at the prospect of a journey across the city. The ambulance to take me to the hospital arrived as I was finishing lunch and the whole ward wished me success. It was a fine day, the sunshine reflecting my mood. Would my surgeon recognize the progress which I saw? He did. 'Put the little finger of your left hand into your right ear.' Oh, I was so used to that one it had ceased to hold any real significance! The first few demands I achieved with ease, then he produced one impossible request after another. It was like a pin in a balloon. He checked the state of my scar infection and expressed concern. I explained that until my mother's devoted attention at Christmas it had been far worse. He thought for a brief space and then prescribed daily application of silver nitrate stick, explaining its function. He would see me on February 10th when, if I had progressed sufficiently, it should be possible to start planning discharge. There was a glimmer of light at the end of the tunnel and I rejoiced.

Knowing that it would be some time before the ambulance returned, I managed to fit in a visit to the Social Work department and then to my old ward. There I had a rapturous welcome from Sisters, staff and therapists. What they had achieved through me was almost inconceivable. I had survived odds of ten to one and had proved myself not to be a permanent invalid. My success was theirs. All their dedication and bitter effort had been rewarded. Back in the rehabilitation hospital, my tea had been kept hot for me and people were eager for news. That evening, in a rush of enthusiasm, I began drafting a letter to my parents to tell them the good news. It took me two days to write. 'Dear Mum and Dad, News! I saw my surgeon on Monday and he thinks that I may be ready for discharge in a month. I see him next on the 10th February; the decision will be taken then. He was optimistic about my chances of being discharged then.' In a day or so they also received a letter from my surgeon in which he expressed pleasure at my progress: 'She is walking very well and the right arm is improving all the time. Her spoken speech is still very hesitant but she is now writing with great facility and at a high level indeed.' My parents were delighted with the news but even more so that, in all his volume of work, he had taken the time and trouble to write a personal letter.

Life went back into its normal routine. All too soon the physical benefits of my Christmas week were a faint memory. I clung to it, struggling against the exhaustion of an intense schedule and inadequate sleep. One day, during the brief respite between the end of lunch and the beginning of afternoon therapy, I was lying on my bed listening to the sounds of bustle in the ward kitchen along the corridor. There seems to be a ritual in hospitals that the clearing away and washing of dishes is accompanied by the maximum amount of noise, as though to say, 'We're working. How about you?' There is something comforting about the sameness of it all; the clamour, the clatter, the shouting. By contrast the ward was quiet; sedate, peaceful, civilized. Suddenly at the other end of my bed, strung between the curtain surround and the ceiling pole, I noticed a large cobweb. It was extremely dusty, for it had been the reflection of light on the dust which had first drawn my attention. It was so fine, yet must have been there for months to collect so much dust.

Diana, in the bed diagonally opposite mine, noticed my rapt expression and asked its significance. She followed my directions and located the web. Her horror was not that there were spiders, but what the age of the web must signify about the cleanliness of the ward. A couple of days later, she pointed it out to the cleaner. Usually good-humoured though the cleaner was, the result was an explosion; invective flying about in all directions. She 'hadn't got time to sweep cobwebs off of rails and anyway what did we think she was?' And she 'was damned if she was going to climb on a chair and take a broom to anything'. Jokingly next day Diana told the only staff nurse on the unit, who shrugged her shoulders, but after being reminded of the cobweb's presence every time Diana met her, eventually she swept it down. I was slightly sorry to see its demise; it had been there so long that it had become part of the scenery.

The Sisters tried to maintain a good standard, but they were fighting a losing battle. I estimated that there were about four unqualified nurses to every qualified nurse of any rank. On one particular occasion, a rather harassed Sister had to manage for two hours on a double ward of sixty patients with just one auxiliary nurse. The night staff were a different story. Except for one SEN covering the double ward and a touring Sister covering half the hospital, night staff were all auxiliary. Not only was it difficult to reduce their noise level, but some of them were completely unable to visualize how they would feel in the same situation, and appeared deliberately non-cooperative. Their self-defensive blindness made me angry. All my hard rehabilitative work accompanied by inadequate sleep and utter exhaustion was beginning to have disconcerting effects upon my personality. I became increasingly short-tempered and my tolerance decreased sharply. I was very unhappy to see these traits developing, but was loathe to divert precious energy from my recovery on to the niceties of polite social living.

Progress in physiotherapy was very slow. My therapist and I would put in days of intense effort to reduce paralysis or release spasm with seemingly no result. One day Miss Appin went out of the gymnasium for a few minutes, leaving me weight-bearing on my right arm. I practised. It was excruciating. Every second my arm was yelling at me to stop the agony. Fleetingly I relaxed, but the thought of being left for the rest of my life in my present disabled condition heaved me back to the bar. 'Think of something to take your mind off it.' I could manage a few seconds mental release, but then the pain would come roaring through. Involuntary tears rolled down my cheeks. Guessing that they would not be the last, I didn't bother to wipe my face. 'Divert your mind!' But however I tried I could not get away from the pain. I was only sustained by the knowledge that Christ shared my pain or rather that I shared His.

Trying to have a satisfactory wash was difficult, my feet and legs being the greatest problem. I soon began taking a chair with me into the curtained cubicle, which ensured that I was that much nearer the ground should I topple. One evening, wrapped only in a towel, I was busy washing my feet. I leant forward to gather more soap and as I did, the chair slid from under me, backwards through the curtain. I lurched to the right, banging my head with a noisy crack against the lockers, and slumped in a naked heap on the floor. There was immediate panic on the other side of the curtain: 'Nurse, Nurse!' Don't worry, I thought, it's happened before. My legs from the knees down were now protruding from beneath the curtain. I began to try to get to my feet, to be abruptly brought to a halt by a panicked voice from outside.

'No. Don't move.'

I heard a nurse rushing down the corridor. She appeared discreetly round the edge of the curtain to be greeted by my naked figure, smiling beatifically. She drew back in horror.

'What are you doing there?'

I didn't bother to answer as the question seemed rhetorical.

'How did it happen?'

Briefly I explained that I had been washing my feet and had lost my balance.

'Washing your feet!!' exclaimed the astonished nurse as though it was the first time she had heard of the practice.

'Get dressed and come back to the ward.'

'Not until I've cleaned my teeth,' I said, struggling to my feet.

Not long after that incident Sister Hood offered me a bath. My enthusiasm surprised her; I could not have been more pleased had she offered me a crock of gold! The offer was repeated the following week. What bliss to feel totally clean. One of the auxiliaries grumbled to me that other patients had to wait longer in between baths. I defended myself by saying that last week's bath had been my first. Sister Hood and I were developing a warm relationship based on the fact that

I made no secret of my understanding of the difficulties under which she worked. We discussed my permanent tiredness and she agreed to do what she could.

By this time my written language was becoming more fluent. Mrs Macfarlane made good use of the progress in the exercises which she set me and I positively revelled in the new developments. One Friday afternoon she set my homework for the weekend: 'Write a description of your favourite character from *The Canterbury Tales*. No Chaucerian English, thanks.' It would not be a case of my favourite character, but simply the one about whom I could remember most! With some sense of achievement, I submitted on Monday morning: 'Chaucer: The Prioress. Chaucer pokes fun at her but he is not cruel; we laugh with her rather than at her. She thinks of herself as speaking French well but Chaucer comments that it is after the fashion of Stratford-at-Bow – in other words her French was catastrophic! She has never been outside England, but likes to pretend that she has. She likes to keep up appearances and Chaucer comments about her foot attire not being quite regulation, but highly fashionable. She gives herself airs and graces.

Chaucer points the finger at her not in judgement, knowing that she, like so many others of her time took the veil to be secure and independent – not for the right motives. Life in a convent had not subdued them. She is sentimental without being constructive and it is with kind yet firm irony that she has hanging from her waist the quotation, "*Amor vincit omnia*".' Beware those who had implied that this haemorrhage had terminated my usefulness!

Most paramedical therapists will support patients and gladly carry them through the inevitable times of exhaustion and depression, while the patients replenish their strength. For this they have to make an agreement, often unspoken, that when their strength is replenished, they will shoulder the burden themselves. At the time, it may seem that the task is unsurmoutable, but it must be tried. The temporary transfer of responsibility may last a couple of minutes, hours, or days, but both carrier and carried know that the patient will eventually take up the burden again. When it is properly used, it is one of the most precious aspects of caring. It has to be a conscious, shared decision. An ultimate achievement programme has to be set.

It was lack of recognition of the need for a planned, shared programme that caused so many patients to stagnate, progressively to diminish their activity and their personality and retreat from the struggle. A few reached the stage of being little more than bodies to be fed and watered at appropriate hours, whose sole conversation had become platitudes and minor grumbles. They had only themselves to blame. I found eventually that I regarded as progress the most seemingly minor developments such as the first time I managed to construct and deliver a grammatically correct sentence, instead of a string of related words. I was so excited that I promptly stumbled over the next sentence. That didn't matter, the important thing was the achievement.

Suddenly, in the last week in January, I was transferred to the single room adjacent to the ward. Although it was closer to the kitchen than my bed in the ward, an extremely heavy wooden door reduced the clamour to a faint hum. Inside, the room breathed peace. I was overjoyed. Here I could relax, work and sleep undisturbed. I expressed grateful thanks to Sister Hood. Here I was sometimes forgotten by nurses and slept on in the morning undisturbed until half-past seven. After three or four days the benefits of more sleep were clearly visible. I became less taut, less contained; more expansive. My stifled sense of humour and warmth to other people blossomed.

One day, soon after I had changed rooms, the Principal Social Worker from the previous hospital came to see me. She had brought with her the last slip of my salary entitlement. She apologized for the lateness of its arrival and hovered as though uncertain how to begin. Of course the hospital were concerned and I wasn't to assume that I'd been sacked, but it was administratively convenient to terminate my contract. So, staff can be laid aside for 'administrative convenience' can they? So much for Department and Health Service care of employees. I had long since realized that immediate return to my previous appointment would not be feasible, but had hoped that until a return to practice was possible, that I might have been appointed to a tenable clerical post. I'd worked against the odds rehabilitatively, hoping that return to work in some field might be possible before dissolution of my contract became necessary. They might at least have waited until I was out of hospital. I was angry that they'd been too cold and blind not to foresee the inevitable blow to personal determination and integration which simultaneous announcement might bring. My superior was now describing how praiseworthy the Board of Management had considered my work and that she was sorry to be losing such a good social worker. With bitter, defensive irony I said, 'Oh, really!'

She looked up, surprised, paused for a few moments and then choosing her words carefully, seeking the least incriminating, said that the Board wanted me to know that when I was ready for work that they would consider any application from me favourably.

'Right. I would like that in writing please.'

The blow to my determination was enormous. I had been laid aside like a used rag or a spent match. Had I enough strength to fight against the assumption that my useful days were over? I did not know. The only thing I did know was that I certainly was not over! For a few days even my little room somehow seemed less important, except as a place where solitude was to be had. This was no good! I vigorously pulled up my socks. To integrate this type of experience positively into your personality and to progress towards health, you need confirmation that *you* as an individual have not been diminished. This was what the hospital and society through fear, short-sightedness or incredulity was not prepared to give.

The general public is afraid of what exposure to the disabled is going to mean for them. Fear of abnormal limbs, the assumption that speech defect equals brain defect, the automatic conclusion that acceptance and involvement with the disabled is going to damage those who expose themselves, only emphasizes the division between the disabled and the rest. I decided that the least I could do was to try and wear down public ignorance, avoidance through fear and the patronizing attitude which lays an added weight on the shoulders of the disabled. I decided to stand firmly in society's firing line and withstand those who denied my capability and considered me superfluous. Example speaks louder than volumes of theory. Did I have the strength? I did not know, but somehow, deep down inside, my intuition told me that I did.

January crept on towards my next clinic with my surgeon. Both Mrs Macfarlane and I were hoping that he would consider discharge feasible, so she began exposing me to various normal, everyday experiences. She made me practise talking on the telephone. At first she would begin talking before introducing me. Then came the day when she just handed me the receiver with the phone still ringing. The call was to Elisabeth at the general hospital. I managed, but only just. I found it extremely difficult to cope with people whom I could not see, particularly people I did not know. I was afraid about what they might think of me. At least when I could see people I could gauge their reactions, but I couldn't do this on the telephone. The tonal contrasts in my voice had been flattened which made verbal gradations almost impossible.

In consultation with my other therapists, Mrs Macfarlane planned outings from the hospital in order that I might try out independent survival with her support. During some excursions I began to realize that frequently it was not I who could not cope, but other people who could not cope with the challenge of me. It was their defence to treat me, despite the contrary evidence, as though I was half-witted. On the second excursion I was brought face to face with the horrifying reality of inflation from which I had been protected during the previous six months in hospital. Everything had increased in price, but not the gentle increase I had been expecting. Simple necessities had doubled in price; coffee had trebled. The shock was profound. With the recent substantial increase in the rent of our flat, I did not see how I could afford to survive. Mrs Macfarlane saw me go white and sway on my feet, and taking me back to hospital made me coffee to counteract the shock.

Now I was continually fighting a malaise of inactivity. Even my little room offered scant compensation. I was now sleeping well, but for what? From habit I refused to capitulate, and struggled half-heartedly on. My parents came north again on February 8th bringing my brother with them. It had been a well-guarded secret and I was delighted. Proudly I showed them my little room. But even their presence could not remove my forlornness for long. I felt useless; a chronically expensive piece of flotsam. Why ever had God allowed me to survive? I answered my own question. It was vital to give me fresh leverage, that I satisfied my surgeon's expectations at the clinic. Otherwise I saw an extremely black future.

Monday dawned bright and clear, and after lunch the family arrived in the car to take me to the clinic. Almost at the beginning of the check-up my surgeon began discussing discharge. My mother had extracted a promise from me that I would tell him how unhappy I felt in the rehabilitation hospital. In view of his suggestion about discharge, I was loathe to hazard it and perhaps prolong my sentence, but a promise is a promise, so I spoke. As it turned out, he was very pleased with my confession and said that if I hadn't soon told him, he would have wondered whether I was abnormal. He said that he would advise the rehabilitation hospital that I was now ready for discharge. It would take several days to come through but I should be out of hospital by the end of the week.

He also asked whether I would like to return south with my parents for a couple of months. The idea was very attractive; two months with them and no domestic worries, compared with straight back into a flat and a full domestic schedule. However could I say that I was worried that if I went south my place in the flat might not be there when I returned, and that I would be left homeless as well as disabled? In Edinburgh I would have little chance in my present condition on the open accommodation market. Besides, I was afraid that my drive towards rehabilitation might slow down in the comfortable environment of home, and that I might find myself a permanent resident where I had no friends of my own age. So I chose Edinburgh, saying that I would go south in a couple of months when I had established a rehabilitation schedule. It would be very difficult, but the alternative would be worse. From the insidious decline in my morale, it was vital that I be discharged. Ten weeks of gruelling therapy in difficult surroundings were taking their toll.

I returned to the hospital, and my parents returned to the flat to spread the good news. Jane, however, was surprised as she had imagined that I would be virtually recovered by the time I returned. That evening she expressed some apprehension about the degree of looking after I would need to my mother who sought to reassure her. The following day my parents returned to England and my discharge came through. Had it come before they left, I would probably, despite my arguments, have gone with them; but it didn't. I telephoned Jane at work, in itself quite an achievement because it meant going through two switchboards. The hospital was prepared to discharge me that day providing people knew I was coming. Jane's reaction was not enthusiastic. She was going south for a few days and Pauline, one of her friends, was using my room. We finally settled on my discharge on Friday. The nursing staff, when they heard, were displeased. I was blocking a bed. I telephoned my parents to say that I would be discharged on Friday. The two days passed quickly, helped by all the preparations which I needed to make and by some of the nurses who treated me as though I didn't exist. On Thursday I went around thanking the people who had helped me in making my time in the hospital one of marked improvement. I had come there hardly able to put several spoken words together correctly and was leaving talking in sentences; I had arrived not able to write logical English and was leaving writing paragraphs which could grace any sixth form school book. I would be working with Mrs Macfarlane when arrangements about my out-patient schedule had been settled. The people whom I was most going to miss would be Sister Hood and Miss Appin, my brilliant physiotherapist who had expended so much effort to extend my range of movement. Together we had achieved considerable success.

Friday arrived; I packed my case and put my other belongings together ready for the ambulance. It arrived just before lunch. I collected the discharge certificate for my doctor, said a few hasty goodbyes and departed on the next stage of my adventure. I had been in hospital one hundred and seventy seven days: one working week less than half a year. As the ambulance swung through the hospital gates and headed north across the city, the air held the sweet scent of freedom.

CHAPTER THIRTEEN

'Children of Israel are never alone'

Complaining bitterly about the stairs, the ambulance driver carried up my luggage. I wished for his sake that he had been more perceptive; had he foreseen my struggles up and down those stairs in the coming months, he would have complained less. We found the keys and I thanked him as he opened the door. He stayed just long enough to see me into the hall and then scuttled away downstairs.

I closed the door, leaning back against it with relief, pushing twinges of fear and loneliness to the back of my mind. Going into the kitchen, I looked for a note of welcome and some instructions about what was available for lunch. There was nothing. Of course, Pauline would not know about our customs. I toured each room looking for some indication that my arrival was anticipated, but there was nothing. I tried hard not to think of what my response would have been, had a flatmate of mine just been discharged after six months in hospital.

Feeling hungry, I turned to the fridge. It was virtually bare. I tried the cupboards; there was a reasonably generous assortment of tins, all too large for one person. Not knowing what our relationship might be, I was unwilling to jeopardize it at the outset. I might inadvertently eat our supper. Returning to the fridge, I helped myself to the only egg and a couple of slices of bread. Taking a jar of Marmite from the cupboard, I sat down to my first meal at home.

Pauline returned late, in a hurry because she was going out with her sister that evening. She had eaten in the middle of the day and was simply going to have tea. She hadn't expected to feed me and asked what I had been doing all the afternoon. Hadn't I thought of going shopping? I choked back the tears and tried to say that I hadn't realized that it would be expected, blurting out that I was too scared. In the ensuing silence, I asked if she would help me to make a temporary bed. I had tried during the afternoon and had failed.

After tea her sister arrived, taking care to keep well clear of me as though I were dangerous or contagious. If it hadn't been so tragic, it would have been funny. The two of them went out. I knew that I must not let myself go. I desperately wanted to have a good howling cry, but could I retrieve myself once I began? Even God seemed further away. As an antidote to rising despair, I eventually telephoned my parents, walking backwards and forwards in front of the phone until I had enough courage to use it. My father's voice at the other end of the line was like melted honey. Thankful of his proffered support, I stumbled through the events of the day, leaving nothing out.

When Pauline and her sister returned later that evening, I was considerably more stable and accepted the news that she would be moving out the following day with equanimity, if not relief. With remarkable forcefulness, I found myself saying that I would only agree to them breaking the contract with the hospital if Pauline would come shopping with me in the morning and would help in the remaking of my bed. The meekness with which they agreed surprised me. Later that night I sat thinking. I had really been thrown in the deep end; a case of sink or swim. It was all up to the Lord; I knew that alone I didn't have a hope. I smiled. Providing fear was not allowed to get a grip, the next few months should be exciting.

The following morning, going down the hill towards the shops I was very nervous, thankful that Pauline had agreed to come. My legs shook with fear and my stomach felt like water. I headed for the shop where I would have to do least talking, thankful for these days of supermarkets. Halfway through Pauline excused herself and went off. When I emerged, she was nowhere to be seen. The most difficult shop remained, a greengrocer's with the traditional counter. Well, there was nothing for it, we needed the food. Praying and rehearsing in my mind what we needed, I went in. Nothing had changed, the piles of fruit and vegetables, the queue, the earthly smell. 'Hello', said the assistant as I reached the counter, 'haven't seen you for months.' 'No', I replied, 'hospital. Brain haemorrhage', as though that explained everything. The assistant screwed up her nose and expressed concern. What had it done? I indicated my right arm and said, 'No speech.'

The assistant was very patient while I said the things I needed. Generally shopping was a nightmare, not only because of my lack of speech but also because of problems of managing existing shopping, the purchased article, purse and change, all with one hand. In this shop it was different, they seemed unconcerned about time and although very busy, helped me stow my goods. Feeling a little more confident, I emerged on to the street. Pauline was nowhere to be seen, I headed for home. Although I had bought just enough for the weekend and Monday, I found myself struggling, exhausted, upstairs, one flight at a time.

Pauline returned with her sister and brother-in-law early in the afternoon, and after a lengthy moving-out process, the last carload was packed and they were gone. In her inability to cope emotionally with my situation, Pauline had been expecting support from me. The expectation, which was to become familiar in future months, was a shock. For the rest of the day I pottered about, trying out the methods of tackling domestic tasks which I had been taught in Occupational Therapy, getting a glow of pleasure with each success. Although far removed from the idealized setting of the Home Unit, here the same methods were still applicable. I accepted the challenge to my ingenuity with delight. With daring I lit the water for a bath and attached my bath-aid to the taps. Hopefully, this would allow me to bath independently. I had tried it in an empty bath at the Home Unit, but the real testing time would be now. I wondered whether I should wait until there was somebody else in the flat to whom I could call in an emergency. I looked thoughtfully into the bath. The room had a party wall with the flat next door and Mrs Smith had a key to our front door. If anything happened, I could hammer on the wall as a distress signal. I knocked on the door and explained what I was planning to do. The bath was a lazy, luxurious delight and, thanks to the Lord's vigilance, passed without mishap.

Jane arrived home the following evening. I was intensely relieved by her return and tried to express my added delight about life, simple everyday events which had taken on a new significance. I failed miserably. I was unwilling to ask for anything beyond what she offered. I had been hoping that she would volunteer to cook for the first week, while I settled into an Out-Patients' routine. She didn't, so I cooked, consoling myself with the thought that she would be cooking next week, which according to my speech therapist would be more difficult than this. With disappointment which sometimes bordered on despair, I discovered that my fairly respectable cooking had tumbled from its pedestal.

It was virtually impossible to judge cooking times correctly and serve constituent parts of a meal fast enough for nothing to spoil. What had been a source of great pleasure became a nightmare. I had never realized in how many procedures I took two mobile hands for granted, like straining vegetables which now became a complex procedure with the colander in the sink. If I served one vegetable first, it would be virtually cold by the time that I had the next one off the gas. Finally the main body of the meal could be rescued. Sometimes in the middle of this procedure, I would call to the drawing-room for aid and rescue and Jane would appear to cope with the removal of a casserole or pie, or on Sundays to carve the chicken or joint, which I massacred with one hand. My one consolation was that my cold desserts were as good as ever.

One evening shortly after my discharge, my mother telephoned and Jane answered. Before calling me I heard her say: 'She does her turn at cooking and everything gets done. I don't know how she does it.' I noted it with mixed feelings. The silent struggles were to be a prophecy for future months.

I began attending the rehabilitation Day Centre at the hospital on the Monday after my discharge, being collected and returned by ambulance. The mornings were very tiring as I instinctively tried to crowd a day's work into half the time. Sometimes as I drove myself onward, I wished that the quest for improvement was not so automatic. Other patients took their progress much more casually, frequently giving up when not under the therapist's watchful eye. I pressed on, and began to find patients talking about my courage. If they had seen the cowering wretch whom God was supporting, the 'me' who was frightened that my progress would stop before I considered survival acceptable, they would have changed their minds. I condemned myself for my lack of faith. If the Lord allowed my progress to cease, He would have good reasons and would provide the necessary support. I should be able to accept whatever level of disability God chose in the same spirit of rejoicing with which I had stared at death, but I couldn't.

On the first Wednesday I had an appointment with my general practitioner to bring her up to date with my progress. I supplied her with a resumé of my hospitalization and told her of my out-patient schedule. She examined my scar and we discussed its perturbing nocturnal leakage. Since my discharge I had been cleaning it every morning with disinfectant solution. She prescribed Hibitane solution for cleaning. I had signed on to her list three years previously, when I ceased to be a student, and had consulted her infrequently. Our rapport had been immediate. My surgeon had indicated that I would be on my drugs semi-permanently; I was worried about financing my prescriptions. Unless I could be supplied with massive prescriptions, I would need to apply for economic exemption. My doctor explained that Epanutin, which she had prescribed, is one of a special category of drugs; by applying to the Executive Council I should be able to get an exemption certificate. I was very relieved, but said that I would try the Department of Health and Social Security first; if I qualified on economic grounds, it would automatically open the doors to rent and rate allowances and a number of other benefits. It turned out that I had just above the maximum level of savings, but I smiled down the telephone receiver at the abusive assistant who told me the news, and contacted my GP, who set the wheels of the Executive Council in action.

I could only walk well over short distances, after which my right foot dropped, dragged and my balance became unsteady. I found the large step on to Corporation buses a mountain climb and the problems of getting on to pay-as-you-enter buses with money ready, were enormous. The easiest way to climb aboard was with the fare clamped between my teeth. To keep my walking to its optimum, I had frequently to catch buses, preserving precious strength. It was a terrible drain on my meagre income. I had to limit the social life which I so badly needed, in order to eat in the middle of the day. I discussed with my doctor the validity of my applying for a Disabled Person's Travel Permit, which if granted would give me free transport within the city boundaries at the wave of a pass.

My Sickness Benefit expired in the last week of February when I was transferred to Invalidity Benefit. I was a little perturbed about the name, which had an unacceptably permanent ring. I calculated that after rent, gas, electricity, telephone, television, stair and general housekeeping fund, I should have £2.75 a week to cover everything else. We each funded our weekday lunches from our individual purses; at weekends they came from the housekeeping. My first reaction was that with a fair drawing-in of the belt, I would be able to manage without dipping too far into my so-carefully accumulated savings. It took all my Benefit merely to survive. It would take weeks to save up for shoe repairs; those shoes which, with my uneven gait I wore out, I did not have the money to replace.

All too soon I found myself in a financial strait-jacket, as month after month my application for rent and rate allowance failed to be granted. The worry was significantly slowing my progress. I was reluctant to use my savings because I knew that once touched, it would be like a drip on a stone. One day, feeling particularly pressurized as quarterly bills were pouring it, I withdrew a hundred pounds from my share account. The feeling of economic relief was intense, but the rot had set in. It was to take a year's struggle and another disaster to overcome this need for some financial security.

There is something far wrong when a state encourages people to save and then penalizes them, if they become ill, for having taken its advice. The Welfare State is run at the expense of the lower-middle and the middle class; by this I mean those who are aware of tomorrow and have a disposition to save. People like myself who, through age, illness or unemployment come into long-term contact with the machinery of the Welfare State find themselves at a real disadvantage.

From their thriftiness and propensity to save, they find themselves penalized by the system. Often, having followed the State's encouraging advice, they will discover that their savings are above the allowed limit, with little or no realistic guarantee that when their savings have fallen below that level, their application will be given credence. Benefit rates are deliberately kept behind the rate of inflation. Thereby the government saves money, but those least able to withstand it, the old, the disabled, the unemployed, are penalized. The costs in human anguish are incalculable.

I was coming to know several of the ambulance drivers by sight. I enjoyed sharing their open friendliness, watching with an appreciatively professional eye the way they dealt with their passengers. On one return journey from the hospital I was collected by a particularly friendly, jovial driver. As yet I was his sole passenger. He swung his ambulance with gay abandon in front of the building. Inside I clung grimly to my seat. Realizing that I could not avoid slipping, I tried to call. No sound came. I toppled to the floor, giving my head a noisy crack on the floor. The ambulance driver made an emergency stop which would have gained credit from any Ministry of Transport examiner, and came anxiously back down the ambulance. I was shaken and mildly concussed. I wanted to go home, to have a cup of coffee, and to gather my shaken wits together in peace and comfort before starting to prepare the evening meal. It was my cooking week.

The ambulance driver in his anxiety had other ideas. He drove me around to my old ward and spoke to Sister. As the accident had happened in an ambulance, I would have to be X-rayed, to compare with previous plates for evidence to disprove additional damage, in case I decided to go to law. Nothing was further from my mind. The ambulance driver was a kind man and I knew that it would be a long time before he would be absentminded again. I was anxious about getting home to cook; my relationship with Jane was deteriorating and I could not afford extra problems. No choice was afforded me; feeling very frustrated, I asked Sister to telephone Jane to explain what had happened and what was available for dinner. When a radiographer at last arrived I was taken to the X-ray department in a wheelchair, although

I was quite capable of walking. It was the reverse of all their usual practices. As anticipated, the X-rays proved clear, after which I had to wait for an ambulance to take me home. I eventually arrived about ten o'clock.

As the month ground on towards the time when my parents would be coming north to fetch me, my spirits sank and my frustration grew. I desperately needed someone who had the strength and perception to see the inner, basically unchanged me: the superstructure of my disability blocked everyone else's vision. They looked at the disabled person in front of them and failed to realize that I was still the same person behind. My comprehension was normal even if I spoke in grammatical shorthand. I didn't want to be avoided or held at arm's length. I needed acceptance and integration.

Everybody wanted to share in the successes; few friends had the perception and the courage to share in the grinding misery of defeat. None of these few were available except on a very irregular basis. Mrs Macfarlane saw me on weekdays, but there was so much work to be done that there was often little more than a tacit recognition that the problems existed. In my need, I began building a reserve support fund into which I gathered whatever a person was capable of giving, and manipulated myself into using this to its fullest, rather as deprived children, at untold cost to their personalities, manage in residential care with a whole regiment of inadequate substitutes.

Although I only saw him intermittently, one friend, Simon, was a pillar of strength because he was prepared to accept me as I was. A group of friends, feeling guilty for their lack of contact during previous months, took me to an opera. I absorbed their concern thankfully, like parched ground soaking up rain after drought. There were a number who invited me for coffee, sherry or a meal. For some it was a way of apologizing for having doubted my survival. What I found hardest of all was that I was being used by a group of neighbours as the latest topic for gossip. Yet they meant well, so I smiled and said nothing. One of Jane's friends offered me a ticket for *Joseph and His Technicolour Dreamcoat*. I could not afford it but I needed the encouragement, so I went. One sentence was brought forcibly home that night, never to be forgotten: 'Children of Israel are never alone.'

During the month I tried to think through the reasons why some of the experiences in hospital, of both staff and patients, had been so positive and others negative and utterly destructive. I had regarded the experience as an exciting opportunity to share in an undefended way the very stuff of life. How much learning had taken place depended to a great extent on the response of the other person. In the face of defensive, self-protecting reactions by others, I would find myself automatically less willing to share. Early in my illness, when I realized what was happening, I tried to stop the temptation to respond neutrally as a method of avoiding confrontation. That was simply doing what they were, and I would learn nothing that way. Rejection is costly, yet the staff and patients who were prepared to use their own personalities undefendedly in their work or rehabilitation had far more positive experiences than those who sat stolidly behind the protective defence of their professional roles.

Many people use their professionalism as an excuse for non-involvement, a disguise for their reluctance to share. They are frightened of being hurt, of having to maintain clarity of vision through untold personal pain. They hold themselves back, not realizing that it is they themselves whom they are holding at arms' length. In the days of my pre-professional practice, my insecurity had made me afraid of challenge and I had worked with an invisible protective wall between myself and the people whom I was sent to help. During my professional training I had squirmed to think of the additional distress I must have caused some of my early clients. But that was exactly what I had seen in some interactions around me during my hospitalization. It produces a vicious self-propagating spiral of tension and fear. For the positive survival of patients and staff, it has to be recognized and surmounted. In the second hospital it was the fear of losing their viability, in a complex profession which they little understood, that made many auxiliary nurses respond so negatively. Trained staff were scared because they were vastly outnumbered by auxiliaries. In their defensiveness they could

108

not see that it was their own personalities which were being twisted and destroyed.

The central problem is that amongst all their other learning, people have not been allowed and taught to explore their own reactions to trauma. Experienced professionals under emotional pressure start to feel uncertain, strained and, because the symptoms are unfamiliar, 'unprofessional', they feel insecure. They begin to wonder, like Dietrich Bonhoeffer, 'Am I that which other men tell of? Or am I only that which I myself know of myself?' Doctors, nurses and therapists each spend years learning the technicalities of their profession. Learning to cope with and integrate the personal stress involved is scarcely touched.

All of them should have a period towards the end of their training when they learn about personality structure, when they have the opportunity to look into themselves with help and guidance. They should be helped to face their basic mistrust, shame, doubt, guilt, inferiority, isolation, despair and role confusion. With perceptive, supportive help, they should peel back the layers from the onion of their own personality. During the psycho-dynamics course of my Social Work Diploma, I had been exposed to such a programme. It had been hard and emotionally painful to face myself, stripped of illusions. I had dragged up from the murky depths facets in my personality of which I had only been subconsciously aware.

They needed accepting, incorporating, integrating, developing, so that the knowledge gained might be used to help me recognize where my own life experience would significantly affect my approach to a situation and to estimate the degree of significance. Overtly recognizing what caused me stress, anxiety, joy, fear, helped me in understanding and accepting the inner, unspoken needs of others.

The length and intensity of courses should be geared to the requirements of individual groups. Untrained auxiliary staff should have an introductory, possibly in-service course in which simple nursing techniques are explained and where they are introduced to the concept of using heightened awareness of themselves, their patients and colleagues, as a standard practice. Although it requires additional expenditure, it will soon be more than recouped in improved staff welfare and increased patient progress. Staff frustration, patient isolation and delays all mean money. Patients would become actively involved and work towards their own recovery, enabling faster discharge. This would mean greater turnover, less bed-blocking.

Fear is the root of all evils. It is through fear of non-acceptance that people disguise or deny their own needs, sometimes even to themselves. In the hospital setting it manifests itself in rigid maintenance of rank, and by staff demanding that patients respond as their inferiors. The Big-White-Chief syndrome, prevalent in many hospitals, is not an acknowledgement of learning, but an expression of insecure power. Real security is expressed in a willingness to share. Mutual knowledge of our ultimate security in Christ, whatever happened, was what had made my conversations with my surgeon so open and positive. It was this which made the nursing nun such a perceptive friend to all. She treated every patient as her equal, knowing that but for the grace of God she might be one of them. The response which her undefended openness achieved from other people was incredible. Awkward patients, valiantly disguising their fear, would suddenly melt in the warmth of her non-judgemental understanding and would return care and thanks.

Patients who hardly share a word with their consultant beyond, 'Yes, sir', will happily talk to cleaners, because they feel of similar status. The result is that much helpful, revealing information is lost to those who need to know it. Patients are often afraid that their fears will be taken for negative criticism or ridiculed. It is easier to express them to equally unknowing patients or domestic staff, which gives the temporary relief of physically talking, but leaves the original anxiety still unresolved. Sometimes it appears in physical symptoms, baffling to medical practitioners because they seem unrelated.

People's subconscious imaginations are capable of producing horrors far more devastating than the truth. The shunt was a prime example. I found patients using me as a listening ear because I accepted them and their fears. If the question was something which I could not immediately answer, I would suggest that they asked their surgeon, Sister or social worker. I knew that from a hospital bed it was easy for me; I didn't carry the can. Yet I did share in the responsibility for those asking and the quality of the response. I felt the same degree of concern for the surgeons as for the patients. For my own surgeon I felt even greater concern because of the openness of his response. He had been risking his career on me. It would have been far easier to have looked at me in Casualty and said, 'No hope.' But he hadn't, he clutched at a straw and it had held. He was aware that my social work insight helped me to know more than he told me verbally, that I recognized what he did not say as if he had said it. Apart from my need to know, openly recognizing that my survival was unlikely had made me attempt to share the responsibility for the operation. If I had died, at least he would have known that I had remained enthusiastically supportive. My decisions about the quality of my life or death had been partly intended as a compliment to his courage.

CHAPTER FOURTEEN

God had Other Ideas

I gave my notice to the ambulance service and my advance April rent to Jane. My parents came north to collect me. It was comfortable and secure waking in my old bedroom, listening to all the familiar noises downstairs, knowing that there would be hot water and breakfast without my doing anything about it. But however great my relief at escaping from the suffocating atmosphere in the flat, and no matter how comfortable I was in the south, if I was to achieve anything like a normal life, I had to return to Edinburgh to continue my treatment. We cleaned my scar in the mornings, reserving physiotherapy sessions for the evening.

Feeling brave one evening, I telephoned Sally, an old schoolfriend who had married a vet and had a ten-month old baby. Her response to my abbreviated language was an enthusiastic invitation to visit them. Panic rose from my stomach to my throat. I dearly wanted to see them but I was frightened of the journey and of their reactions. How would they accept me? For almost the first time the easiest way seemed not to find out. I thought of all the negative reasons I could, including the problem about travelling. Could I cope with the trains, the London Underground, escalators, a case, crowds? Sally told me the times of the trains and that she would be at Horsham station to meet me the following Monday. I would return on the Thursday. The telephone went dead. Help! What had I done? I had a violent urge to phone back and chicken out.

My father took me to Victoria Station and I bought my ticket. The clerk, mistaking me for a foreigner and talking painfully slowly, volunteered the platform number. I found a suitable carriage and swung my case in. The tread between the platform and the train was so narrow, and the step between the platform and the train so deep, that it caused a problem. If I put my left leg on the step, the distance between the platform and the train was too great for my right leg. I was unwilling to try it the other way round, or to put both feet on the step, because of its narrowness and Southern Region's electrified lines winking at me through the spaces.

Finally I put my strong left foot on the step and raised my right knee far enough to kneel on the floor of the carriage. I hauled myself inside in an unladylike manner, thankful that I'd chosen an empty carriage.

Sally was at the station to meet me, her usual, bubbling, cheerful self. She had little Elizabeth in the car with her. It was the first time I had seen my future goddaughter. We returned to the house and, for the first time, I knew the frustration and maternal yearning of seeing a small child in front of me raise her arms to be picked up and of not being able to do so. I could have managed with my left arm, but undoubtedly she would feel insecure with so much space around her and would find it frightening. It would be answering my needs, not hers. I could form the sort of relationship she would need by playing on the floor with her. At last I found someone for whom my language was totally adequate.

With Sally I knew the frustration of only being able to say a fraction of what I wanted. I longed to share something of the incredible depth I had discovered in life, that if you suffered alone it was your own choosing because no matter how deep you went, God could always go deeper. I had discovered that once you had learnt to accept, you always had support. I had known this in theory for years; now I knew the reality. But the chasm between thought and language was so vast and it took so much effort and single-minded concentration, that it ruined any attempts to converse at that level. Sally's husband, Alan, accepted my lack of spoken vocabulary as though it didn't exist, and encouraged me to expand my thoughts in the relaxed atmosphere of their home. I began to develop simultaneous prompting techniques which, although slow, enabled me to conduct a more fluid conversation. It was the first time since the operation that I had been able to achieve two things simultaneously. Jubilant, I shared a little of the sudden release with Alan and Sally. It

113

still required a conscious effort to verbalize, but if I really concentrated I could think about speech production and follow a topic at the same time. A gag had been released.

In the evenings Sally and I got down on the carpet to do my physiotherapy exercises. Acting as resistance and leverage, she was fascinated, and competing against each other we frequently dissolved into gales of laughter. For those few days time lingered: quiet Sussex villages, the ploughed fields, circling birds, friends and firelight in the evenings, gentle laughter. Winter was holding its breath, watching, waiting for the beginning of spring. The expectation of new life seemed an allegory of my recovery. The impossible almost achieved. But my progress was like a drip on stone: I felt so active, so alive on the inside, but desperately hindered by the restrictions my body placed on me. If only I could shed it and indent for a new one. My brother, south for Easter, drove down to collect me. I had glimpsed again what life could be and I wanted more. As we travelled home, as though warning me not to expect too much change in my situation, it snowed.

Three weeks slid gently past. We went to the Ideal Home Exhibition and ordered my washing machine. I visited several of my parents' friends to thank them for their concern and to let them see the extent of my recovery for themselves. Their reactions spanned the whole spectrum from those who were openly prepared to recognize what had happened and shared the uncertainties and rejoicing with me, to those unable to accept being faced with events which they did not understand, who treated me with kid gloves. The self-preserving reaction of 'Never mind, dear', like 'Does she take sugar?' is damaging because it is, unwittingly, subhumanizing. There were those who had known me before my haemorrhage who, because of my exterior limitations, now saw me as blighted and impoverished. In their fear they failed to see the in-built strength I had gained from experience. I felt some sympathy with them but saw that in protecting themselves they were not only isolating me, but also themselves.

It had been agreed that I should come south for a month. I had been in England for almost six weeks. I had made considerable progress, but it was vital that I returned to my therapy schedule so that the improvements could be consolidated. The thought of Jane surviving in domestic isolation made me feel guilty. I telephoned to tell her the date of my return, and that I would be seeing my surgeon the following day. But when we arrived and were taking my luggage up the stairs, she looked askance at the cases and later asked my mother: 'Why all the cases? Is Kristine staying here?' My mother explained that my therapy schedule would restart, at which Jane expressed surprise. No comment was made about my progress.

When I went to the hospital for my surgeon's clinic, I was enthusiastically welcomed by the nursing staff, acclaiming my progress. The immediacy and warmth of their response was a great encouragement. The feeling that they knew some of the cost of progress was in itself a support. My surgeon expressed guarded pleasure at my progress, but concern about the continuing infection. He discussed possible courses of action, saying that he would check its progress regularly for several weeks. As a last resort he would have to take me back to theatre and scrape the bone.

I returned to my therapy schedule, enjoying the amazement expressed at my progress. Mrs Macfarlane and two occupational therapists told me that even being optimistic, the most they had anticipated was that my capabilities would not diminish. Instead, I had improved dramatically. They asked what I had been doing. I explained how I had come downstairs in the mornings to find a pile of exercises waiting for me: language from my mother, which I enjoyed; maths from my father, a penance completed in order to secure the promised calculator. I told Mrs Macfarlane how I had frequently longed for the simplicity of her basic arithmetic.

The response of the hospital to my improvement was to cut my schedule from five half-days to three half-days. My first reaction was, 'Is this how they repay me for all my hard work?' I was beginning to fall into the trap of resenting the removal of help when I was working so hard. Briefly I wondered how many people, if only subconsciously, have been discouraged from progressing because they knew that when they did, the help would be withdrawn. Now, when I could cope with more, was precisely when I should be driven harder. I knew that recent patients needed basic treatment more than I did, but while I was still economically unviable, I was loath to reduce my rehabilitation programme. I upbraided myself for being unrealistic and decided that if the hospital were going to diminish my therapy, I would assist my continuing progress by enlarging my other activities. I discovered that the bookshop in St Giles' Cathedral needed a helper on Thursday afternoons. My speech was still grossly inadequate for this kind of work, which mainly involved talking to visitors, but it would be something to keep my mind alert and hopefully improve my speech.

As my beautiful, sultry-skinned occupational therapist, Jenny, watched me weaving and carpet-making she issued a heavy challenge. Now my speech had improved, I should write a book. We had begun discussing some of my observations and ideas about staff and patient perception before I went south. She had been very enthusiastic. But when she had suggested that I put my story on paper, I had replied that it was beyond my capabilities and it had been left at that. Now, in the light of my improvement, she was more determined. She produced arguments to support her idea, telling me that I was in a unique position, with experience of the situation from three sides. I was a patient, an employee of the Health Service with perceptive knowledge about the problems faced by medical staff, and I was a practising social worker. Had there ever before been somebody more qualified to comment on the total situation? The question was rhetorical, but it stung. I could see the implications of her challenge and knew that I should respond but, quite simply, I did not have the strength. My constructed language was so poor. Although ideas·came easily enough, simple paragraphs for Mrs Macfarlane took me ages to produce. Frequently my present memory was not good enough to retain complex ideas, while I manipulated language into acceptable sentences. The main barrier was frustration: I knew it and my inability to conquer it made me more frustrated. At present I simply had not enough strength to face up to the challenge, so I warded Jenny off with platitudes. However, God had other ideas.

One afternoon in St Giles' later in May, I was approached by the editor of the 'St Giles' News', the Cathedral's broadsheet. He asked me if I would write a short article about my illness, what had happened, how I had reacted and what the experience had taught me. I backed away; I couldn't. My language was too poor, the barrier between thought and writing still too large to bridge. I was about to answer no, when it occurred to me that this might be what God wanted. If that was the case, I would have to do it. God would provide the words. I hesitantly agreed to try, warning the editor not to expect anything publishable. Was God really asking me, or was it merely coincidence? The answer would lie in whether I was able to write anything good enough or long enough to warrant publication. That evening I planned structure, and made notes. To my surprise I discovered that I knew what I should write. The problem would be whether I could produce enough acceptable sentences. I went to bed that night with an uncanny feeling of excitement.

The following afternoon I settled with my notes. Now would be the real testing time. If the flow of thought and writing came readily, I would assume that my writing was God's intention. If it didn't come naturally, I would stop. 'The 26th of August 1974 dawned like any other summer's day.' I set the scene of my collapse, and went on from there, astounded at the ease with which it rolled on to the paper. I tried to explain the post-operative horror of discovering that I couldn't speak. 'My silent world threw me almost completely on to the strength of God. In my outwardly speechless world I talked more than I had ever done with God, in my head. I hope I also learned to listen more too. I learned to share absolutely everything with Him. Before, I had been apt to share my life with God, but I expected to be responsible for most of the little things myself. Not any more. I let Him run everything now.' I continued about the long uphill road of learning to speak again, and what the experience had taught me about learning to cope with my own failures and frustration. 'I have grown more tolerant with myself. I have learned to let myself get away with the things God lets me get away with.' That was bad grammar, a preposition at the end of a sentence. But no matter how I tried to reconstruct the sentence my mind was a blank; so it was left. I continued up to the present, and ended, 'I have been given the grace to share a little of the agony of the cross.' No, despite its truth,

I couldn't write that. People would misunderstand. I finished much more lamely.

I was amazed that, with my notes, I had completed it in an afternoon. As I read it over, I discovered that I was unable to produce constructive criticism. I was able to see the faults, but had no idea what to do about them. That evening I gave it to a friend to read, to get a realistic criticism. She read it, saying 'I never realized' and 'I never knew', and gave it back with great enthusiasm telling me not to alter it, not even the mistakes. I handed it in on Sunday and waited for the reaction. A few days later I was told it would be printed in the June issue. I suddenly became scared and felt indefensibly exposed. I had put my soul on paper and it was going to be printed for anyone to read. We had a large congregation and copies were always left at the doors for visitors. It was the beginning of the tourist season, so there was no telling how far it would reach.

CHAPTER FIFTEEN

'Hard pressed, but not crushed . . .'

Over lunch the following week, Jane said that she thought it would be better if we stopped sharing the same flat. She tried to keep her voice level and calm, pointing out that three years was the longest she had ever shared a flat with someone before. Although I had been expecting something of the sort for weeks, the reality was like ice down my back. I disregarded the temptation to retaliate, fighting down the insecurity rising somewhere between my stomach and my throat. 'Don't panic, don't panic!' The social worker in me was pleased that Jane had summoned the courage to say in the open what had obviously been brewing for months. To retaliate would only be to rub salt in an open wound.

Realizing that I would have to answer, I chose the least expected route. I spoke of my pleasure that she had, at last, managed to verbalize her anger, insecurity and frustration, and explained a little about the dangers of suppressing important emotions. This gave me time to assess my capabilities for coping with an unknown move, or a prolonged wrangle.

I had moved into the flat in 1971. The arrangement had worked well. I gave Jane my rent in advance and she paid the landlord. He preferred it that way because it meant one cheque instead of two. It had never occurred to me to have my name added to the tenancy contract. I had grown very attached to our Regency flat and was loath to move out, but something would have to be done.

I knew that I did not have the strength to face the competition of the open market. To face unknown flat after unknown flat, trying to sell myself as a potential flatmate: if I put my energies into that, my rehabilitation would grind to a halt until I was resettled. It could take months and I did not have months. Every week counted; my rehabilitation was a race against time. So I spread the word among my friends and acquaintances in dancing, church and social work that I needed alternative accommodation.

My cooking week began the following Saturday. I had organized for myself a rota of local shops as my days of bargain hunting elsewhere were over. I would walk down the hill and shop on the way up. That meant by the time I reached the butcher's and my left arm felt as though it had reached my knees, I was nearly home. This particular Saturday the shopping bag felt heavier than ever. The paralysis unbalanced me at the best of times, but with a heavy shopping bag on my left arm which I was unable to change, it was much worse. I climbed two flights. There was one more before I reached the first flat; ours was two storeys above this. My arm was aching so much that I rested the shopping beside my feet when I reached the top of the stairs. It began to totter. 'Ah! the eggs!', I thought, as I lunged at the bag. I saved it, but the sudden movement had so unbalanced me that I started to fall. Realizing what was happening, I tried to grab the banisters and missed. With startling clarity of thought, I turned over on to my back in mid-flight and remembered to relax. I landed at the bottom of the stairs with a painful thud and gave my head a noisy crack. It seemed to jar every bone in my body.

My first reaction was to get up to my shopping and pretend that nothing had happened. I wriggled my toes on my left foot. Theoretically there should not be any spinal damage. But I had lain quite still since I had landed and it was going to be very difficult to get up. You had to laugh. I was lying resplendently, flat on my back, with my body at the bottom of the stairs. My feet, trailing above me, were automatically at ninety degrees, from years of country dancing. If I had cracked a vertebra, trying to get up on my own would inevitably break it. I listened. I could hear people in the flat above me. I called for help several times, but there was no reaction. The only other possibility was to call Mrs Smith, my disabled neighbour on the fourth floor. Remembering that people can hear their names when just out of earshot, I used the echo of the stair well to call, 'Mrs Smith, can you help, please?' I heard her door open. She called: 'Kristine! Where are you?'

I explained what had happened, and heard her coming down stairs with her stick at a violent pace, hammering on doors as she passed. Other neighbours joined her, and as they turned the corner above me, gazes of horror met my broad smile.

One neighbour immediately dashed upstairs for strong black coffee as an antidote to shock. I sipped it thankfully. There was a general decision that I ought to be X-rayed, and another neighbour offered to drive me to hospital, while Mrs Smith was left with instruction for Jane about what was for lunch. At the hospital shots were taken of my head and spine; there was no damage. Following the fall, the borehole leaked blood for about ten days, frightening me until I was reassured by my surgeon and doctor that it was quite acceptable. On my return, a neighbour whom I hardly knew after four years of living on the same stair, asked me in. She asked about my shopping and whether Jane could not come with me. After I had explained that we shared cooking and housework equally, this neighbour offered to take me with her in her car every other Saturday. Although she went to a more expensive area, I accepted gratefully, and it worked well for the first two occasions. On the third she sent a message that she would not be available and on the fourth, although she took me, she seemed to be regretting her hasty enthusiasm. She never offered again.

Later in June I was again approached by the editor of 'St Giles' News'. He had decided I ought to have my copies before my article was published. He said that, as a doctor, he had been fascinated by the account and would like to meet me sometime to hear more, particularly of the problems I had found in personal rehabilitation. As well as sending copies to my parents and my brother, I gave one to my speech therapist as an encouragement for her work and another to my surgeon for information. And the next time I went into St Giles', the usual piles of the newsletter were at the doors. I quietened my rising sense of isolation, the fears of having put information about my inmost being on paper for the world to read. Well, if that was what the Lord wanted, it was all right by me. Although I might feel exposed and lonely, He would provide support. After the service, people gathered round me expressing their congratulations, thanks, amazement, encouragement, concern, interest and support. It was almost as though God were saying, 'I told you so.' The next time Jenny urged me to write a book, I agreed to try.

On the 6th July I was comfortably settled in my armchair watching television, when a peculiar flashing started in the right half of my right eye, regularly twice a second. I ignored it in the hope that it might go away. After several minutes vivid memory flashes started, also in the right half of my right eye. They were so real that I kept turning my head to see the image more clearly. The images, alternating with the flashes, were fascinating. The first flash had almost frightened me. It had been of Harry, seemingly right beside my ear. Instantaneously I had realized that it was an image because I could see too much of him from where I was sitting and I also recognized the scene from last summer's holiday. The recalls were completely haphazard, scenes from early childhood muddled with recent events. I tried to watch the flashes; they were like round multi-pointed stars. Some of the points at the right-hand edge seemed to disappear beyond my eye into my head. Automatically my eyes followed the image round, forgetting that it would remain constant because it was happening inside my head.

At this stage the incident did not particularly worry me because I thought I knew the cause, imagining that it was a mild epileptic-type fit. My surgeon had explained that I would have to remain on medication semi-permanently to suppress the likelihood of my sustaining an actual fit. His words went through my mind now: 'After much extensive brain surgery it is only to be expected.' But after several minutes of combined flashings I was feeling very sick. I stood up to rush to the safety of the bathroom, only then realizing how unsteady I was. Lurching drunkenly towards the door, I staggered into the hall heading for the bathroom, only to find myself opening the front door. Virtually blind from the flashes, thoroughly disorientated and now very frightened, I eventually found the bathroom, only just in time.

Jane must have heard my mad, erratic dash around the flat. I tried to call reassurance and an explanation to her. Not a sound emerged! I tried again; something indistinguishable

122

came. When she appeared in the bathroom doorway, all I could say was 'flashing' and indicate that it was my eyes. She went to fetch Mrs Smith and, as neither had any idea what was happening and I was unable to say, they decided I should see a doctor. As I was due for a check-up with my surgeon the following day, I reckoned there was little that could be done but, being in no state to argue, I acquiesced.

To my horror I discovered that my speech had regressed six months in the space of half-an-hour! Surely God didn't intend me, having come so far, to retrace all that slow, agonizing road again? If that was the case, I would be much better giving up the fight. It was made worse because I knew that it was not in my nature to give up; I knew that I would be a stubborn pig-headed fool and plod on regardless. Hot tears of exhaustion and frustration welled up and overflowed. Six months' hard work for nothing! When the doctor arrived there was, as I had thought, virtually nothing he could do. When he asked about my next appointment with my surgeon, I managed to say 'Tomorrow'. He did what he could in the situation by giving me some anti-sickness pills and ordering me to bed.

The next morning my speech had regained about two months on its performance of the previous evening. I spent the morning compiling a record of the evening's events, painstakingly producing a version of what had happened for my surgeon. The frustration and distress of trying to write caused burning hot tears. My mother's warnings haunted my mind: if I drove myself too hard, I would make negative progress. That was exactly what had happened. Once in my surgeon's room, I passed him the note. He read it, smiling and nodding, and asked me to explain in my own words. I began. I knew what I wanted to say, but it came out sparsely and all jumbled. The desolation was incredible and there was my surgeon sitting in splendid isolation behind his desk, nodding and smiling broadly! I could have shaken him.

Seeing the scowl of disapproval on my face, he began to explain. The experience was known as a 'Todd's Incident' and was caused by a sudden distinct burst of healing and tissue growth. As I began to relax, he went on that this particular development was probably in the part of the cortex

123

at the back of the skull, which controls sight. He was, however, particularly interested in the alternating memory flashes and their vividness. This was far more unusual, indicating either two separate incidents or that the second was triggered off by an overflow from the first. During the conversation, he enquired whether I had ever suffered from migraine. I said that very occasionally I had a headache severe enough to make me sick. The flashing, he explained, was a more common form of migraine. Side effects could be any combination of nausea, vomiting, loss of balance and complete loss of concentration.

He clipped my note into my records. I looked at the terrible scrawl and felt dreadfully exposed. But it was an explicit demonstration of what had happened and needed to be said. He saw the direction of my gaze and explained, with something approaching tenderness, that it was important as a record and that it wouldn't be looked at negatively. My speech and writing should return to normal within a few days and subsequently I should notice a distinct improvement, surpassing the pre-incident level, in both my speech and writing ability. Breathing a huge sigh of relief, I therefore ceased to worry and everything turned out exactly as he predicted.

CHAPTER SIXTEEN

First Anniversary

In July the ambulance service stopped transporting out-patients to therapy sessions as a form of industrial action. As Jane passed near the rear entrance of the hospital, she agreed to give me a lift. From where she left me, the way to the Day Centre lay through extensive grounds for about a quarter of a mile. The view was incredible. Large conifers framed glorious expanses of Pentland Hills. 'I will lift up mine eyes to the hills,' I joyfully proclaimed to squirrels quietly breakfasting under the trees. 'From whence does my help come?' Then exuberantly repeating the psalmist's answer: 'My help comes from the Lord, Who has made heaven and earth. He will not let your foot be moved, He Who keeps you will not slumber.'

Mrs Macfarlane worked at my comprehension and writing speed, giving me dictation, comprehension and grammar exercises. I supplied subordinate clauses, imperfect indicative and subjunctive verbs in assorted cases, pluperfect and past historic; each demand became more complex than the last. To try and conquer the hesitations and silences we repeated nonsense rhymes: 'The common cormorant or shag, Lays eggs inside a paper bag,' and 'The dreadful things that rabbits do.' I practised rhythm at home, using anything that came to mind: hymns, poems, 'The Twelve Days of Christmas', 'Green Grow the Rushes', Gilbert and Sullivan slowed down. Gradually my speech was becoming more fluid.

In Occupational Therapy I had been making a rug from string and wool. As I had become accustomed to the technique and lost interest in the pattern, I found myself doing it without thinking. In a few weeks I had doubled my speed, but was automatically developing substitute techniques as it failed to grip my interest. One day Jenny found me admiring a patient's painting in the workroom. Could I draw? I ad-

125

mitted that I had been considered quite good at school. With relief, she found a draughtsman's board and paper, and told me to choose my own subject. I went outside and helped myself to a stem of roses, laid out the arrangement, collected pencils and rubber, marked out the spacing guidelines and began carefully to draw.

Seeing the unseen, I began to build up a rose. Gradually it became not just a rose, but a specific identifiable rose. It gave me a sense of security; at least this talent had not been lost. As one rose became two and grew stems, patients came to see how the work was progressing.

'With your left hand too?'

'I've always been left-handed.'

This seemed to increase their amazement. I heard women further down the table talking in hushed whispers. 'And she draws with her left hand!' I smiled at their ignorance.

Jenny was impressed and suggested that if I didn't get back to my profession, this might prove to be alternative work. I looked at my drawing with surprise. It was a fairly good amateur piece of work, because the art master at school had taught us to interpret three-dimensional structure on paper, and I had a keen eye and a steady hand; but to break into the world of art was something I had never considered. If my speech did not improve enough to allow me to work in the community, it was definitely an avenue to be explored.

Since late May, I had been editing and extending the new edition of the information handbook of the Scottish Council for Single Parents. I had come to know the Director during my years with the Guild of Service. She knew that I maintained information files on a large number of benefits and facilities and had requested my help. In her office I shared the frustrating tale of my application for Rent Allowance. Early in the spring I had applied, and had followed this up with several enquiries which had been answered with 'under investigation' and one 'no record'. By mid-June I was thoroughly disillusioned. My rent was just over one third of my Invalidity Benefit, without gas, electricity, telephone and food. The next time I enquired, I asked whether the procedure was really so complex that it took three months to decide whether someone on Invalidity Benefit qualified for a Rent Allowance.

A week later I was sent two sets of forms asking for evidence of Jane's income as well as mine. The accompanying letter implied that our incomes would be assessed jointly and then halved. Apart from the fact that I had no idea what Jane's income was, there was no reason why they should know. I returned the forms and wrote a letter which ended by stating that Jane 'is not and cannot possibly act as a philanthropic institution'. It was followed by yet another silence during which I had to pay another month's rent, the renewal on my insurance premium and a telephone bill. Julie-Ann suggested that I apply for a grant to the Social Workers' Benevolent Trust. We worded the application together.

Meanwhile a wonderful possibility began to fill my mind and lighten the load of worry. The Dunedin Dancers had been planning to send a team to our Austrian friends. Although I could not dance, I could not contemplate their going without me. In spite of all the odds being against it, I longed to thank the Austrians personally for their concern, and to show them my progress. Most of all, I wanted to prove to myself that I was still capable of maintaining a positive role in a group. The news went round the neighbours like fire through tinderwood and I was stopped on the stairs to be lectured on my lack of realism.

I was due to go south to my parents for a holiday, my surgeon having been assured that the department of industrial physiotherapy at Hawker Siddeley would accept me for therapy. The day before my parents arrived to collect me, final confirmation of the trip came through. I decided to write to Harry to ask for his honest reactions to the possibility of my coming and to find out whether, if my surgeon should grant permission, the team's doctor would be prepared to have me as a member of the group. The Scots had meantime agreed, providing I had my surgeon's permission. Then came Harry's enthusiastic reply, and I wrote to my surgeon.

At home I spent a lazy fortnight visiting neighbours, reading and relaxing. Then the dream of floating gently through the summer was shattered at the news that the physiotherapist from Hawker Siddeley Aviation was expecting me for assessment. But in spite of my trepidation at this new adventure, it was clear within a few minutes that Ann and I would get on well, and I was soon exercising independently with rope and weights. I liked the blunt way Ann introduced me to the first batch of curious patients: 'She's Reg Gibbs' daughter.' Acceptance secured, I enjoyed the way she unobtrusively stimulated the men to encourage each other. At the end of my first morning we planned four sessions a week for four weeks.

These weeks at Hatfield provided the opportunity for me to explore the feasibility of Jenny's challenge to write. My partial paralysis was diminishing, but my speech was still very limited. The responsibility of the task and my lack of ability weighed on my mind. My father's colleagues were, however, intrigued by the idea and I was allotted an office and facilities within the Personnel Department. Each morning I would have physiotherapy with Ann and spend some time wired to a Farradic Oscillator, then I would phone across to my father's office on the other side of the airfield. In fine weather I would begin walking around the perimeter track to meet him. The rest of the day would be spent writing, and talking to people who were concerned and interested.

I relaxed into a soporific routine in which I was not required to make any decisions beyond what to wear and what to have for lunch. After this, returning to independent living would require so much effort, hard grind, frustration, rejection, defeat, that it would be far easier just to give up. I was sure that Hawker Siddeley would find me a small corner doing something innocuous. My parents, sensing my retreat into safety, suggested I should move home with them again. The offer was tempting: to put an end to all the struggling, to go home and float through life. But I would be going home an invalid, defeated by the challenge of recovery.

I was shaken from my lethargy in the middle of August by a letter from my surgeon.

Dear Kristine,
Your letter arrived when I was on holiday and I hope it is not too late therefore to answer. There is absolutely no reason why you cannot go to Austria with the dancers and

I hope you have a jolly good time. I am delighted to hear everything is going well.

I read the letter again and again, scarcely able to credit his optimism. The phrase 'jolly good time' echoed in my head. What a statement of confidence! 'Do you really want to go?' my mother asked cautiously. 'Of course!' I said, every vestige of defeat suddenly vanishing.

That evening I telephoned Christine Taylor, the Dunedin secretary. Outside the medical profession I could count on one hand the families who were fully prepared to recognize that my thought processes were normal and that I was not of diminished responsibility. The Taylors were one such family. The rest did not mean it unkindly, but what I needed was positive not negative support, the expectation of success, not failure. Surmounting the expectation of failure requires more energy, the aggressive attitude of 'I'll show them!', which is much harder and infinitely more wearing. Christine was delighted by the news of my surgeon's permission. The rest of the group already had their tickets, but she was sure an extra one could be arranged.

Then she hesitated before telling me that, as she was going to spend a term on teaching exchange in Grenoble, she wanted to take her car and would be grateful of company on the journey. Would I consider driving with her? The opportunity seemed too good to be true, and I agreed enthusiastically. When she reminded me of the long hours in the car, I replied that the car would be carrying my case, that I could map read and my knowledge of local roads in Austria might prove useful. She had booked a cabin on the overnight crossing Hull to Rotterdam, and there should still be enough time to book the other bunk in the same cabin for me. My parents were very pleased with the arrangement and my father immediately said that he would finance the ferry. I did not then know that Harry was to offer the same generosity for the journey home.

Everything dovetailed with incredible precision. Planned months before, my parents' holiday was the last week in August and the first two in September. My August clinic with my surgeon was for the 25th; Christine and I would leave for Austria on the 28th. I would return on the 7th of September.

129

Even our arrangements for the Edinburgh Festival fitted. And when we arrived at the flat on the 24th, a letter was waiting for me from the Social Workers' Benevolent Trust. 'The Trustees have asked me to say how very sorry they are to hear of your difficulties, and to enclose a cheque to help with your present commitments.' It was for fifty pounds. I held it in my hands, trying to believe in its reality. I had received a week's taxable salary and suddenly felt rich. Automatically I found myself planning what it could do: two months' rent, or one month's rent, the gas bill and a pair of sandals. I wrote to thank the Trustees.

In my mind I had waited with longing for the day when my hair would reach the stage of being long enough to warrant trimming and shaping. Now it was about two inches long, a ragged urchin cut. Before my illness I had not fully appreciated how closely my feminine identity was linked to my hair. When I was bald, even under a wig, I had felt a sense of shame. As I walked into my usual salon, it felt like a triumphal procession. I had not been there for more than a year. The receptionists recognized me and I could feel them looking askance at my hair, thinking 'Who's been let loose on that?' But when I had explained the reason for the haircut and the slow speech, their concern that I should have an experienced hairdresser, as mine was fully booked, was evident. Having booked the appointment, I emerged from the salon as though walking on air.

When my father and I arrived at the Out-Patients' Department of the hospital that same afternoon, it was a hive of industry. Wistfully I looked at my old office door as we crossed the entrance hall. Nothing had changed. Only the faces, similar in their burden of anxiety, were different. Mentally I watched myself emerge from that door, lock it, turn, smile supportively to someone sitting nearby, trying to stimulate warmth and confidence with my eyes. I wondered if any of them remembered. I doubted it. Perhaps somewhere in their subconscious memory it would have lit a little spark. At the clinic I was greeted enthusiastically by the Sister and the staff, remarking on my progress. I felt pleased that they had noticed: it took so much unrelenting effort. My surgeon had been called away on an emergency. When he eventually arrived, striding down the corridor at great speed, there was a crowd waiting for him.

In his office, I was at last able to thank him for the expression of confidence which the letter and his permission had contained. I told him of the success of my physiotherapy sessions, giving him a demonstration of additional movement achieved in the last six weeks, and passed him a sealed letter from my parents' general practitioner. In early July my surgeon had sent him a summary of my recent medical history. As my surgeon read the letter, his face darkened. Despite all our care, the scar infection had erupted again. I had told the doctor that my surgeon was treating it with Ceporex and had requested another course, but he had refused. Instead he had put me on an extremely heavy dose of Sulphatriad. I had pleaded with him to keep to my surgeon's prescription, but he was adamant. He said it was a kill-or-cure dose. Within a few days I was having severe side-effects; nausea, vomiting, lethargy, exhaustion and my vision affected so that I found focussing difficult. After ten days it had been so severe that my father had dragged me unwillingly back to the surgery. I would have tolerated the side-effects for a lasting improvement to the infection. On my father's insistence, the doctor reverted to my surgeon's prescription. When he finished reading the letter, my surgeon looked at my father and thanked him for his action, explaining that had I continued to take that dosage, serious side-effects would have resulted. I did not ask what they were, the tone of his voice was enough.

That evening we visited my speech therapist as she had invited my parents to do so when they were next in Edinburgh. On the doorstep she talked excitedly about the improvement in my speech. 'You haven't heard anything yet', I grinned, 'I've been given permission to go to Austria.' As she had always shown interest in my Austrian friends, I had brought my dirndl with me. She admired the scarlet wool brocade bodice and the black skirt. She was amazed at the fluency of my speech and congratulated my mother on her success. Incredulous, my mother tried to diminish the significance of the role she had played. It gave me great pleasure to have caused Mrs Macfarlane such a profound sense of professional achievement. She had shared the depression, the exhaustion and had given unstintingly so much of herself. I was delighted to be able to return a little of her success.

Tuesday was the 26th, the first anniversary. During the day my mind automatically traversed the year. I wondered if it was abnormal to find oneself following a day so closely. No, not this year, when last year I had not expected to survive. Statistically, I shouldn't be alive and yet, through the grace of God, here I was. I looked down at myself, the strengthening arm, felt the blood pulsing through my veins I might not understand His reasons, but I could certainly revel in His grace. That evening we had tickets for a Festival Concert which included Beethoven's Ninth Symphony. I listened to the words of Schiller's 'Ode to Joy' in the last movement with new understanding. 'Thy power reunited all those whom the world has divided. All men are brothers. Whoever has a soul to call his own, joins the song of praise. Any who cannot must creep weeping away. World, do you know your Creator? Millions, do you worship Him?' We sang the words together as we came out of the concert hall. What a celebration!

After a few minutes I suddenly realized that I was walking and talking simultaneously. A few hours ago I could achieve each individually, but I could not concentrate on two demanding tasks at once. I had often tried, only to find myself grinding to a halt, achieving neither. In the car a three-way conversation developed, which only hours before would have brought a cry of 'Jamming'. We were on the way to pay a quick visit to the leader of the group going to Austria and, as he lived up a dark, old twisting stair, I suggested my mother came with me for the experience. While we climbed, I explained some of the social problems connected with life in crowded tenements. Gradually it dawned on me that I was climbing and talking simultaneously. Not wanting to break the spell, I flapped my hand up and down excitedly. Broad smiles were exchanged; nothing more needed to be said. Good old Beethoven!

On the Wednesday morning my father and I went off to attend to last-minute arrangements. When we returned my mother looked very troubled, almost in tears. At first she was reluctant to tell me, but then said that she had met our neighbour and, regarding her as an old friend, had told her of my progress and the trip to Austria. She had turned on my mother and told her that I should not be allowed to go, that it would be unfair on the people with whom I was travelling, unfair on the Austrians, and that I would overtax myself. She had then gone on to say that I should not be left to friends and neighbours in Edinburgh, and that I should be taken home for protection and looked after properly. The last part was very heavily stressed as though implying that my mother did not want me at home. My mother had explained that my surgeon had not only given permission for me to go to Austria, but had encouraged me to do so, and that from the beginning we had obeyed his instructions implicitly. But nothing my mother said could placate the neighbour.

If she could have seen my mother's battles not to be possessively protective, she would have changed her mind. I put my arm round my mother's shoulders 'If I had been content to be "put out to grass", I would not be struggling so hard for rehabilitation now. Don't worry, Mum. It's just she who can't cope.' I then proceeded to take every one of my neighbour's points and, taking both sides, explained what had happened. I had chosen to remain in Edinburgh because not only was that where my surgeon was, but also my friends and professional contacts. When my therapy ended, I would need work. I had thought very carefully about what I could tolerate on a long-term basis and it would have to be something challenging, stimulating and mentally demanding; otherwise I would vegetate and my survival would not have been to any purpose. God doesn't expend so much energy getting somebody to live, only to have them waste it.

That afternoon I packed and had my long-awaited hair appointment. The reception which I received in the hairdresser's was so openly enthusiastic that it dimmed any doubts I might have had about whether I ought to move south to relieve neighbouring consciences. My own hairdresser came out to meet me; it was a year since we had last met. With great concern she asked how I was and what had happened. Gently and positively, I answered her questions. She was almost crying. I touched her sleeve, 'I'm all right now.' The salon could not have treated me with more consideration or care had I been royalty.

Months before I had arranged tickets for the Military Tattoo for that evening. As I was spending the night before our departure with Christine, we packed into the car my case, overnight bag and the vast store of food my mother had prepared, and found a parking space near the castle. The sea of humanity pouring up Castlehill seemed a little incongruous in anoraks and blankets on a warm summer evening. This was one of the most exciting events of the year for my mother. I watched her unreserved delight with pleasure. At the end of the evening I climbed down from our stand and down the steep, uneven steps steadily in dense crowds, the measured skirl of the pipes echoing in my ears.

Christine and her mother were at the door to meet us and a sleeping bag was already laid out for me on the sofa in the sitting room. My mother explained how our food parcel was packed and gave a little anxious advice. We wished each other happy holidays and my parents arranged to collect me from the station on my return. We kissed, waved and they were gone. During that year they had travelled 14,748 miles between south Hertfordshire and Edinburgh, that is slightly more than a single journey to Australia and a return journey to Moscow.

CHAPTER SEVENTEEN

Austria Again

We left Edinburgh the following morning, reaching Hull in time to board the overnight ferry to Rotterdam and, having slept well, disembarked prepared for the long haul across Holland, Germany and into Austria. By the time we crossed the Austrian border, it was dark and becoming foggy. I gave directions from memory. We reached Route 1 without a mistake and followed the rest of the way as if from habit, passing a solitary street lamp at the corner of Harry's road. It was the first street lamp we had seen since crossing the border. We had travelled 998 miles since leaving Edinburgh and had been on the road for sixteen hours since disembarking in Rotterdam. I rang the bell. On the other side of the door, the dog barked. I called his name and could tell by the changing sounds that he was wagging his tail. Harry's older sister opened the door. '*Entschuldigen, bitte können wir herein kommen?*' With great rejoicing, the door was thrown wide. Harry was away at a conference overnight, but he would be back in the morning.

Upstairs in the vast upper bedroom where I had slept the previous year, I smiled contentedly, thinking of the journey. It had been a minor triumph. Next morning I lay listening to the sounds of the house I had come to love. Short months ago, I had not expected to see it again. I heard the sound of Harry's car outside and then his mother explaining that we had already arrived. As I made my way downstairs, I could still hear the kindness in his voice. I had tried to keep both Harry and his family realistically up-to-date with my progress, but how could I be sure that they would not be expecting much more? As I turned the corner into the kitchen, Harry's answer was immediate and spontaneous: the look of utter relief on his face and his bear-hug of a welcome. The long fight for survival, the months of dragging improvement, the anguish, the exhaustion and the crippling frustration were all worth it for a reception of such sharing.

That afternoon the Scottish group were to be included in the thirtieth anniversary celebrations of the Siebenbürger people's escape from Rumania. This tight-knit religious community had left the persecution and strife of north-west Germany and eastern Holland during the early seventeenth century and had found a peaceful haven in a wooded area of Transylvania. With passing generations the community spread and prospered, but had retained their German language and their religious commitment. With the Russian invasion of Rumania in 1944, those who were able fled, many to Austria. The celebrations were to be a two-day event. Before we left each day, I put my daily dosage of Epinutin into my handbag, guessing that we would not return until late that night.

On arriving in Wels for the celebrations, I received an enthusiastic welcome from the people whom I'd met the previous year. It was not to prove superficial. The Austrians foresaw when difficulties might arise and were always standing ready to assist: when I met with something difficult, like carving barbecued steak, one of them automatically took over, before I struggled and failed. It took me most of the week to accustom myself to the continuous forethought. I told myself on the first Saturday that it was kind and considerate, but that it could not last. By the end of the festival, when it was still happening and I had progressed more than in any week since the haemorrhage, I was glad to admit that I had been wrong. It was the expectation of success rather than failure which made the difference.

That first evening, there was a torchlight procession through the streets. Hundreds of Siebenbürger dancers in traditional costume marched under the arched gate, into the Medieval town square, each man carrying a white candle. The light ebbed and flowed as the dancers performed a vast formation dance, throwing grotesque shadows on the old walls. My eyes blurred with tears. On the Sunday there was another procession and dancing in the park. That evening there was a dinner party for the Scots. After the meal, the dancing began. I had a deep longing to dance, to prove that I was still capable of dancing; that this was not another area of life irretrievably disappearing. Harry asked me to waltz with him. At first I tried to maintain my own balance, then under his gentle encouragement, I began to relax. The waltz became noticeably better. At last I relaxed totally, letting Harry take responsibility for both of us. It was the first time that I had relaxed completely, voluntarily, for almost a year. We smiled at each other, both aware of what had happened, but I little think that Harry realized what a momentous event it was for me.

On Tuesday, after a civic reception with the Mayor, a mountain climb was planned. Rather doubtfully, and under considerable Austrian pressure, I had agreed to join the party. Schafberg, the mountain in question, is over a mile high, but I was assured that the funicular railway stops only a hundred metres below the summit. After a marvellous ascent with glorious panorama unfolding, the time came to dismount. This was the part of which I had been afraid. Suddenly I found two men in Alpine boots at my elbows. Nothing was said about why they were there, but we all knew. When we reached the summit and the two men went off in search of beer, I asked one of the Austrians whether they had devised some sort of rota of people to check and see that I was managing. Her astonishment was genuine and indicated that whatever help I received was spontaneous.

For the next two days I decided not to join the group, but to enjoy the time instead with Harry's family, saving my strength for the long journey home. The last evening was to be our most important performance, in full highland dress, in the main civic hall of Vöcklabruck. I wore full evening dress for my role, front of house. Both performers and audience responded magnificently and the applause was almost deafening, especially for highland dances. As we were to leave for the station immediately after the performance, I disappeared backstage shortly before the end to give myself time to change into travelling clothes.

Suddenly it was all over, the concert, the festival, everything but the goodbyes and the journey home. Until now I had been apprehensive about the journey; thirty-two hours in trains, with several major changes. Now all the anxiety disappeared like a bad dream and I found myself actually looking forward to it. The lights of the train appeared in the distance, the last goodbyes were exchanged, the last promises of return and the train dragged us reluctantly away. After crossing the border at Passau, we made ready for the night. I woke in Frankfurt station at six o'clock. I had slept for six hours. Probably aided by my experience of the atrocious night noise level in the second hospital, I had slept through a ticket check and all the others turning over in a confined space.

We travelled together as far as Dover. I reached Edinburgh alone, after two nights and a day. Punctual as ever, my parents came to meet me at the station: on schedule after nearly a thousand miles. The reunion was a very happy one. The trip had been a phenomenal success, both for the group and more particularly for me. I had received the first positive impression of my capabilities from a group which came neither from hospital, nor from close relatives. I had been accepted just as I was, my personality undiminished, my other disabilities seen as relatively temporary. I now dared to hope that what I inwardly felt was possible and true.

CHAPTER EIGHTEEN

Conference

Now more than ever, I had concrete evidence that the way in which people responded to me was a reflection of their own internal security. Rehabilitation in society, at an acceptably intelligent level, would be possible providing people did not try to exclude me because of their own unresolved fears. In Austria I had received openly concerned acceptance of a kind I had rarely found in Britain. The problem would be how to arouse the confidence of potential employers in my abilities to the extent that they would forget their fears and offer me stimulating employment. That would be my next aim.

We planned to travel south the following day, but first we wanted to take advantage of my new washing machine. As we reached the flat, Mrs Smith was waiting for us at the top of the stairs. 'How did it go?' 'Marvellous, fantastic' I said, launching into an enthusiastic description. She stood incredulous, not knowing whether to believe her ears. Over the months she had been very kind but she too had doubted my ability to cope, particularly with the holiday. As we opened the door, I could not resist saying with a grin: 'And we climbed a mountain!'

I would be returning in three or four weeks, depending on whether or not I was accepted for the Annual Conference of the British Association of Social Workers which was being held in Edinburgh this year. I had written to the headquarters of the Association applying for a grant. I wanted to attend as a way of assessing whether I was still capable of working as a social worker or some backwater of social administration, or whether I would have to look for a new career.

Later in the afternoon when my repacking was completed, a key sounded in the lock. It was too early for Jane. Then I remembered that she had been planning for her parents to visit her. It would be good to meet them. Her father came in with a broad smile and outstretched hand. I responded to his warmth with enthusiasm. When he asked about my holiday, I watched the ease with which precise mental images flowed into words. It was slow, but it was all there in the right place.

When we arrived home after a gentle drive south, a letter was waiting for me from the Social Workers' Educational Trust. The second paragraph said: 'In the past, the Trustees have not felt it appropriate to make grants of this kind, but in the circumstances I will put your request to them when they meet on the 16th September.' The sequel was another letter saying that, 'as a further step towards helping you get back to work' the Trustees were prepared to make a grant to cover attendance for the whole conference; a cheque was enclosed. I made a mental note to seek out the Secretary of the Trust during the conference to thank her for encouraging support. Soon after our return I had a letter from my surgeon, to whom I had written a description of my holiday:

> Dear Kristine,
> Thank you so much for your letter. I am so glad that the holiday was a success. You are doing very well. Keep it up.

This, and the letter about the grant, was so much encouragement that I felt as though I was watching the first glimmers of the sunrise. As we once again travelled north, I knew that how I coped with the conference would decide so much of what would happen in the future.

I had decided to use the day before the conference began to settle finally my application for a Rent Allowance and Rate Rebate. Again I went to the Housing Department seeking news. There was none, only the thickening file of my letters and the vague, diversionary tactics of the counter clerks. Their lack of interest and inefficiency annoyed me. They knew that my income was a standard government benefit and my savings, such as they now were, came well within the limits set by the Scottish Information Office. Why the need for a six-month delay? I left the office angered by the ineptitude of those who administered a well-publicized potentially helpful benefit. Until now I had tried to give the Housing Department due consideration for pressure of work. I could no longer afford to be civil. I walked away, wondering how many pensioners had met with similar responses and then, bewildered and lacking the belligerence to continue, suffered malnutrition and hypothermia in order to pay their rent.

The day before the conference began, I registered and paid my fees, and chose my groups from a selection of over fifty. The theme this year was to be 'Decision-Making in Social Work: Focus on Practice'; I went home with a large folder of material to read through. Amongst the papers was a list of delegates. Perusing it I saw that one-third of my postgraduate student colleagues were going to be present, many of whom I had not seen for four years. Disguising my disability would be a great problem, so I decided to cover up my verbal limitations by remaining a silent participant. Once the conference began, my fourteen-month absence from direct practice vanished into thin air and I found myself responding as I would have in my working days. I sighed with relief: providing I did not try to verbalize, my capacities for comprehensive analysis were undiminished. It was only when I tried to talk or take more than rudimentary notes that I ground to a halt.

After lunch on the second day, the third plenary session began with a talk by Bill Jordan, a figure prominent in social work for his outstanding honesty, on 'Is the client a fellow citizen?' He defined his terms of reference: we all saw our clients as fellow human beings, but did we see them as our moral equals? Did we consider their freedom in the same light in which we saw our own? 'In practice,' he continued, 'loss of citizenship is one characteristic feature of punishments and treatments meted out by our state for deviant behaviour.' I nodded in vigorous agreement. Society defines anything which challenges the status quo, which is difficult to understand, as deviant. This problem had been exacerbated for many by my persistent refusal to collude with their expectations of diminished responsibility. My integrity was too important.

'Do we make decisions about our clients' lives as if they were full and equal citizens, as if to uphold their civil and social rights was to uphold our own; or do we make decisions about them as if their citizenship was of a different, limited kind?' He had hit the nail on the head. That ultimate equality was exactly what I had tried to encourage during my working relationships and had attempted during my hospitalization. If collusion about diminished responsibility, stereotyped ideas about patients not being able to understand, were reduced and avoided, the door would be open for mutual supportive growth. 'It takes a special kind of courage to help clients face the worst aspects of their situation, and of their feelings about them, to share with them their testing of their own resources as they struggle to reach their own solutions to problems.' It is not solely the prerogative of social workers. Conversations with my surgeon prior to the operation had fulfilled precisely this function. It is one of the privileges of sharing in the human condition. When achieved, it stimulates profound mutual learning. Being prepared to risk oneself requires a large degree of internal security. Mr Jordan recounted how, with a client, he had resorted to his knees in a Social Security office. A wry smile crossed my face as I remembered my first interview with an alcoholic recluse, kneeling on her doormat holding her hand poked through the letter box.

That evening no formal entertainment was organized and no-one whom I knew even remotely was visible. Feeling lonely and conspicuous, I wandered from room to room. Before my haemorrhage I would have enjoyed talking to a crowd of unknown social workers, but now I was simply scared of being misunderstood. I hovered on the edge of several conversations, then went into the room where dancing was going on. Theoretically, one day I should be able to sit happily as a spectator at a dance without the urge to join in, but that day was still a long way off. Dancing was too subconsciously entrenched to be relinquished yet and, having lost my speech, I could not help feeling deprived at having also lost my major form of non-verbal self-expression. When I danced my body only succeeded in becoming entangled, as my left side automatically tried to compensate for the paralysis of the right. For years I had been trained to be a dancing perfectionist: I was now an unsteady, clod-hopping hemiplegic.

Leaving the room, I passed a tired man, sitting by himself with his chin in his hands. Neither of us really belonged to

142

the gaiety, and I hesitated, wondering what to do. My first reaction was to join him, but I did not know how he would accept the intrusion. When he looked up, however, I took the plunge, and the warmth of his response told me that I had done the right thing. Brian was an Area Officer from the Midlands. We talked for most of the evening, my speech gradually becoming more fluid.

The next day, the first anniversary of my operation, was also the beginning of the Annual General Meeting. This year one of the subjects for debate was to be the establishment of a Code of Ethics for social workers. The Code would be discussed in the afternoon, and amendments debated. The proposed amendment to Resolution 21 of the Code struck me inexplicably as not quite right. Paragraph 6 in the Statement of Principles stated: 'Basic to the profession of social work is the recognition of the value and dignity of every human being, irrespective of origin, status, sex, age, belief or contribution to society. The profession accepts a responsibility to encourage and facilitate the self-realization of the individual person with due regard for the interest of others.' The intention of the amendment was to have the words 'sexual orientation' added between 'sex' and 'age'.

The intention was obvious. People of male homosexual or lesbian inclinations should be given equal opportunities and not be castigated because they happen to be a minority. I realized that the addition could be positively harmful to the proposers' cause, as everything which they intended was already embodied in the terms 'sex' and 'belief'. Negative criticism was implied by stressing the need for a separate clause. The spirit of the amendment was already in the Code. If the people to whom I spoke at lunch were of the same opinion, the amendment would have to be challenged. I sat next to my former superior from the hospital who agreed with my premise but was unwilling to challenge the amendment. After lunch I explained my concern to Brian who was in agreement, but when I asked him if he would challenge the amendment for me he said, 'No, I couldn't. They wouldn't listen. They'll listen much more to you than they would to me.'

The inevitable was becoming terrifyingly plain. I would

have to speak in case nobody else did. Still I hesitated. Would they listen? Would the trauma of having to speak to a room full of people make my disability worse, perhaps reducing me to silence? Would I make a fool of myself? I realized that this would be relatively unimportant; if I did not speak and the amendment was passed unchallenged, the guilt from my cowardice would live with me for a long time. I didn't expect to influence the result, but at least I would be able to face the amended Code because I had tried. In fear and trepidation, I filled in a form to speak.

Brian and a group of friends escorted me to the front of the hall. As I took the amendment sheet with my little speech to the end of the front row, it felt like the march to the scaffold. I might have experienced butterflies in my stomach before, but this was the first time I had had the shakes. The speech by the proposer of the amendment was brilliant, and I agreed with most of it. I looked for something which would negate the need for me to speak but, if anything, the quality of his speech only made mine more necessary. After the seconder, my turn came. I stood up as my name was announced, went to the microphone, and turned round to look at the sea of faces. My throat was dry and my hand was shaking so violently that I couldn't read what I had written. 'Dear Lord, don't let my speech fail. Justify me.'

I put the paper on the lectern. My vision swam and my knees were knocking so hard that I was sure that people could see. 'Act it, act it.' Straightening myself to my full height, very slowly and clearly I began: 'Madam Chairman and colleagues, I will speak very briefly and I hope to the point.' The room was completely silent, hushed as people began to realize the limitations imposed by my disability:

'I beg to suggest that the very wording of this amendment is, in itself, a form of negative discrimination, by making a specific issue of the sexual orientation differences within our community, for individual members and for the profession. People and members of the profession should be accepted for themselves and their individual qualities without such deliberate clarification.'

Whenever I hesitated or stumbled I could hear people

holding their breath, friends silently urging me on. I gave the room a broad smile. Feeling that I could not go through all the agony of voting, isolated at the front of the room, I made my way back to Brian. Eventually the results were announced; the amendment had been rejected. The proposer demanded a recount, with proxy votes included. Ayes, noes, abstentions and proxies were all collected and collated under the watchful supervision of the Secretariat. Finally the results were announced. The motion had been defeated by exactly one hundred votes. Section 21 of the Code would remain unchanged. I knew that what had happened had great significance for my recovery, but I was too tired to assess it positively.

CHAPTER NINETEEN

'Me again'

Another of the proposed amendments to the Constitution involved the raising of the subscription rates. I did not resent the increase, but it annoyed me that workers earning over £4,000 a year were complaining about having £2 added to their subscription rates, but did not comment on the same increase for workers who were unemployed. There was no time to fill in forms in this case. Very unconstitutionally, I stood and waved my arm to attract the Chairman's attention. She recognized my face from before, and beckoned me forward. It would have to be extempore as I had nothing prepared. Wondering how scared I would feel, I turned to face the meeting. A hall of friendly faces looked back. 'Hello, it's me again.'

I explained that my main concern was that with the increase, experienced members might be lost to the Association. Subscriptions qualified for tax relief, but not if your income was so low that it was not taxable. Surviving on a Government Benefit was no joke. To members isolated through force of circumstances from the day to day life of the profession, the Association and its Journal, *Social Work Today*, were the only means of keeping in touch with current thinking. I thanked the meeting for their consideration when I had spoken before, and continued that I thought they deserved some explanation about my speech. In a few sentences I outlined the events of the previous year and how my perception and understanding had been enhanced.

I said that I would soon be capable of offering the profession far more, but in the interim period before I was ready to work, maintaining contact with current thinking was vital. I had wondered whether to let my subscription lapse when £3 meant so much to me, but a sense of dogged commitment to the task for which I had been trained and lack of relevant alternatives was why I was here today. It was a great concern of mine that in future years when professional social workers of calibre would be desperately needed, no one should have had avoidably to move out of the field. While I had a captive audience I decided to alert their attention to the needs of their colleagues. I had needed guidance about all the benefits to which I was entitled and a social worker who could prevent my thinking round in circles. Having been a source of information for others, previous colleagues were unable to see the sincerity behind the request. It had taken the Association's headquarters, and the Social Workers' Benevolent Trust to respond positively.

Suddenly the bell went for the end of my time allowance. Without realizing quite what had happened, I found myself saying: 'Hey, hang on, I haven't finished yet!' The room dissolved in laughter. They weren't laughing at me, but with me. Smiling, the Chairman signalled to me to continue. I finished talking with considerable problems through my laughter. What a situation! I had stood unconstitutionally, spontaneously back-answered the bell, and I had got away with it.

The Conference finished, delegates dispersed leaving me with an inexplicable sense of optimism. I chided myself; one rose doesn't make a summer. The following week, at his October clinic, I shared the story of my speech with my surgeon, and he was pleased. A few days later I received a letter from the Secretary of the Association who had been instrumental in my attending the Conference. She wondered whether I would be free to meet the Scottish Chairman and herself to discuss the possibility of my manning the Edinburgh office in a voluntary capacity, for a month, until the arrival of the newly appointed Scottish Officer. I was astounded.

At our meeting they outlined their hopes that I would be able to go into the office several days a week, at specific times, to file and re-distribute mail, answer the telephone and deal with enquiries. I was apprehensive and afraid of the responsibility. If I did anything wrong, it might have serious consequences. They assured me of their confidence and that they would keep regular contact. The faith in me was encouraging;

they had more faith in me than I had in myself. It was now or never. It was an opportunity I could not afford to lose. With considerable apprehension I agreed.

CHAPTER TWENTY

The Second Mile

Exacerbated by the strain of my cooking weeks, the relationship in the flat became increasingly fraught and tenuous. My parents, four hundred miles away, found it difficult to understand the depth of Jane's anxiety. My sense of isolation increased, particularly after the Todd's Incident and my tumble downstairs. Neighbours guarded themselves against involvement, retreating behind closed doors as I passed, more frequently than could have been coincidence. I felt sad for them: I understood their fears, but was unable to reduce them. The few people who did accept me became havens of tranquillity in a stormy sea. Now, precisely when I needed more support, the hospital were planning to discharge me from therapy. The unit registrar explained that their resources were limited and that I had already achieved more than anticipated. This I understood, but wasn't stopping my therapy at a point when I was still making positive progress rather premature? Were those at the hospital aware of the other difficulties in my environment? It was agreed that I should be allowed to stay for another month.

The registrar asked if there was anything I needed. Without hesitation I replied: 'Yes, a social worker – someone of calibre.' I desperately needed the support of a professional who could point out the benefits I was missing, who was perceptive enough to analyse the tangled web of relationships, whose vision was clear enough to see when I was thinking myself round in circles, and whose personality was strong enough to prevent my possible manipulation of her. The person would also have to be mature enough to accept working with another social worker. As we talked, one name came repeatedly to mind. Julie-Ann, the Chairman of the Planning Committee for the Conference, would amply fill all the requirements and the registrar volunteered to approach her.

She agreed to work with me and at our first meeting all my doubts about asking someone I knew disappeared in the clarity of her insight. I appreciated her method of working, using herself as a background against which I could explore and expand ideas. She suddenly asked: 'Why didn't you have a nervous breakdown?' The answer was blunt and immediate: 'Because I knew I couldn't cope with one!' Dragged up from the depths of my subconscious, we both recognized its truth.

I doubted whether anyone could fully understand the situation. For several months I had been shielding my parents from the full situation. With sensitivity Julie-Ann explored the reasons why I didn't want to go back to England to live with them. Haltingly, I tried to express the failure which permanent return to their home would symbolize. Neighbours, representing the wider community, would nod their heads and feel justified in their apprehension. I might be down, but I wasn't yet out! I was still hoping some day to return to a branch of the profession or other suitable work. In the south, where law was different, and with a medical history like mine, there was little hope of that. Meantime Jane had asked whether I could arrange an appointment for her to explain her point of view to Julie-Ann. We discussed it and decided that Jane should have her appointment.

Then, one morning in November, my Rent Allowance arrived. It had been backdated to the beginning of June and was for £98.93. After so long I had difficulty in believing my eyes. The Allowance had been granted after twenty-eight weeks. Over the past months I had been learning the temptations of poverty; now the relief was euphoric. I would be able to have my boots repaired, buy some tights and a new jumper all in the same week! My only reckless action, as a way of sharing my good fortune with the world's poor, was to give the whole of the following week's benefit to Christian Aid. I reckoned He'd understand.

Jane kept her appointment. When she returned, she was non-committal but volunteered that they had discussed the problems of living with me at some length. The outcome was that from Jane's point of view it was unsuitable that I should

150

carry on living in the flat, but I would be able to stay until I had found alternative accommodation. For weeks I had been willing this not to happen. Where would I go?

In the quiet safety of my bedroom, tears poured down my face. Why hadn't I died? It was what people expected and would have been much more convenient. Why did homelessness so frighten me? 'He was despised and rejected, a man of sorrows and acquainted with grief.' What right had I to expect anything different? But that night I lay awake long hours, afraid that my resistance would crumble, leaving behind a disintegrated heap of desolation. And when a cheerful letter arrived next day from my mother, something snapped inside. It was my fault for not having revealed the truth earlier. I scribbled a note to my parents, posting it without checking for mistakes. I knew that it would shock them, but it would prepare them for worse to follow.

I was so despondent, so terrified of the problems of the open accommodation market, that I was not at all surprised to hear at my next clinic that my father had written to my surgeon. He in turn had discussed the situation with Julie-Ann, and they had agreed that I was capable of independent living and should be allowed to stay where I would have more fulfilling job opportunities. My surgeon gave me permission to work part-time. To have confidence so positively expressed by a person of his stature was to me affirmation of my worth as a human being. It was two years before I realized that he might have given his permission simply as an antidote to my depression.

By the end of the week I had talked with Julie-Ann, applied for a Corporation flat, had an initial interview with the Disablement Resettlement Officer, met officials from the Disablement Income Group, arranged to meet the Principal Social Worker (Health Services), and bought my rail ticket. My therapy finished on 16th December, and shortly before Christmas I was greatly warmed and impressed to receive a cheque from the Social Workers' Benevolent Trust as a Christmas present. Early in the New Year, the Corporation confirmed that I would be entitled to maximum medical priority and that my Rent Allowance had been at last granted for the previous April and May: nine months after the original

151

application. Slowly I was becoming aware of a new lightness of heart. I ceased to be afraid of misusing my experience professionally and recognized it for what it was, an opportunity to be developed into planned action for others. In discussions with Julie-Ann, we decided that now was the time to get a job which would allow me to move freely back into social work, when the time was ripe.

As though she had heard our conversation, the Disablement Resettlement Officer called me into her office. She had news about work. Exuberantly I went up the hill to the Job Centre. The post was as part-time Assistant to the Assistant Librarian at Moray House College of Education. The enthusiasm evaporated. The post was only during term-time; vacations were unsalaried. This would mean living on Supplementary Benefit during vacations; I calculated that my salary plus Supplementary Benefit would level out over the year to just above my present Benefit. I visualized myself, without adequate stimulation, vegetating in a non-progressive backwater. Would I be required to carry books or climb ladders? She didn't know.

A few weeks later she called me in again. This time the post was at the Royal Edinburgh Hospital. My optimism dwindled rapidly as I heard about the post of filing clerk to one of the research teams. A filing clerk: was it for this I had struggled so hard. Had she a higher calibre of work? I was a graduate and my intellect was still functioning. Her reply was that considering my disability, I would be lucky to get anything. Behind the abruptness caused by having her idea rejected, lay a more serious indictment. She had succumbed to the social doctrine that disabled people are inferior. She was pressurized to place numbers of people; but statistics cannot quantify quality. People became problems to be disposed of as quickly as possible, rather than individuals with unique gifts to offer. As long as the job was physically feasible and socially recognizable, previous aptitude in a different field could be brushed under the carpet.

Increasingly my discussions with Julie-Ann centred on the possibility of obtaining work. The reorganization of the Guild of Service Library was complete. The cross-referencing index, which had begun as a theoretical possibility, was now a functioning reality. In early March 1976, through contacts of Julie-Ann, I was given the opportunity to join a Work Centre for the physically handicapped. The Centre's Social Work team had a job for which they thought I might be suitable. Founded during the last century, the Edinburgh Cripple Aid Society is now more commonly known by its address, Simon Square. One of the many tasks of its Social Work team was the co-ordination of the Disabled Persons' Telephone Scheme. Under this scheme the Regional Social Work Department issue rent-free telephones to disabled, housebound people living alone to alleviate their isolation and enable them to maintain contact with the world outside.

This scheme had recently expanded so much that it required individual attention. As they did not have the finance to pay me as a part-time social worker, I would have to join the Centre as a client. I was to be the link between Divisional Headquarters and the hundreds of disabled people involved in the scheme. It was my job to issue individual accounts, collect returns, answer queries, arrange instalments for people who had difficulty meeting their bills, rectify the backlog, maintain records and organize submission of completed lists and the money to Divisional Headquarters. Twice a week new lists of between 30 and 160 customer accounts would arrive. For my twenty-four hour week, I was paid £2.

I was grateful for the opportunity to be back in a social work environment again, knowing that while I stayed at the Centre, my benefit was virtually assured. It would also give me the opportunity to explore the employment market. Being prepared to listen, I soon found myself being used by younger members of staff as a resource for information and ideas about practice. Once the system was running smoothly, the work was mainly routine, but it felt good to know that my knowledge was of use again. The offices were overcrowded and when it rained the roof leaked, but the cheerful companionship and my joy at being employed again vastly outweighed all other limitations.

In early May the Housing Department suddenly sprang into action. I was called to an allocation meeting about a two-apartment cottage on the south side of the city. I listened to the description, excitement tinged with apprehension. I had lived on my own for short periods, while flatmates were away, but not month after month in isolation, always returning to an empty home. How would I cope? What if I fell? How long would the milk have to sit on the doorstep before help came? Keys were ceremoniously handed over; I heard about rent, conditions of tenure, repairs. Suddenly the official's voice stopped in mid-sentence:

'You can't have this! It's an old age pensioner's cottage!'

She rustled through the papers.

'There's been a mistake. It's marked on some papers and not on others.'

'What happens now?'

'You'll just have to go back on the list.' My heart hit the floor.

'But how long will it be before I hear again?'

'Maybe two months, probably six.'

With administrative unconcern the official was gathering her papers. As far as she was concerned the interview was over. The official put out her hand for the keys. I hung on: possession is nine-tenths of the law. I couldn't let the cottage go without defending myself. I still had their initial allocation letter at home. I asked how their action would stand legally in the eyes of Simon Square or Citizens' Advice? My throat went tight. Although I fought it, suddenly I burst into tears. Oh damn! That was the last thing I wanted! I was angry with the department for having allowed their mistake to slip through two official allocation letters. How, I enquired, would the Minister for the Disabled or the newspapers react to the information that, having sent two allocation letters, the Edinburgh Housing Department were changing their minds because of an administrative error?

Unable to cope any longer, the official left to seek support. Perhaps, after all, the tears were not such a mistake. She returned with her senior who treated me like a naughty child and explained that pensioners were a priority category for housing.

'Do you mean to say that the disabled aren't?'

'But this is a pensioner's cottage.'

'In that case it will be eminently suitable because many problems of the old and the disabled are the same.'

Acutely embarrassed by my continuing presence and my tears, they conferred together. I began to realize that if I stayed there long enough, I would win. The senior official left the room, then returned to announce that as a special concession the Director of Housing had decided to confirm the allocation. I relaxed my grip on the key.

Silently I repeated part of Psalm 86:

I give thanks to Thee, O Lord my God,
with my whole heart,
and I will glorify Thy name for ever.
For great is Thy steadfast love toward me.

In getting me to cry against my will, God had arranged the house which I so desperately needed. As St Paul said: 'In my weakness is my strength.'

CHAPTER TWENTY-ONE

God's Servant First

The cottages, sitting snugly between apartment blocks, were obviously a planner's attempt to integrate the elderly into the community. I found the one allotted to me and looked at the overgrown garden, the broken slates. A useful handrail stood beside the front steps. Inside, the cottage had the smell of a neglected museum. It bore the marks of the solitary old man who had previously lived there. The kitchen was filthy. A thick coat of brown fat clung to the wall where the cooker had once been. Bare wires protruded from the sitting room walls. The ceiling rose hung at a drunken angle; in the bedroom it was a gaping hole. The paper on every wall was torn, stained or dirty. Apart from essential repair work, the whole place would have to be scrubbed and redecorated. On the Monday my father flew to Scotland on business. We spent our brief time together taking measurements, and estimating quantities of paint, wallpaper and curtaining.

My savings had become so depleted that I dared to approach the Supplementary Benefits Commission for help towards essential furnishings. I had a little furniture left me by relatives and had gathered an ample collection of crockery and kitchen equipment. Now I needed the very basics of survival: a bed, gas cooker, wardrobe, chest of drawers, floor covering. However, commission officials said that as I had not been receiving an allowance before the allocation, they could not help. My savings were permissible for an ordinary allowance, but not for a special needs allowance.

As I could not afford to pay double rent, the four weeks before I moved were a race against time. They were also an adventure. I dug into the remains of my savings, deciding what I needed as against what I wanted. While I supplied the cleaning materials, parties of my friends became paper strippers, paint scrubbers and tile washers. Ex-colleagues lent buckets, ladders, brooms, scrapers, scrubbers and a vacuum cleaner. Energetic friends with knives scraped the years of fat from the kitchen wall. Each evening became an impromptu party with people singing lustily as they worked, while I fed them with coffee, milk, soup and biscuits. At the beginning of the second week, electricians removed the wires dangling through the sitting-room walls, plasterers replaced ceiling roses, and I bought decorating materials.

Since early in the year, I had been a member of a small group of Christians from a broad cross-section of city churches, who run Edinburgh's 'Charisma' Folk Club on Friday nights. An outreach mainly by example, it provides a warm welcome, good secular music, good food and an environment inviting open discussion. Before the club opens the team meets for a meal, bible study, song and prayer, and so becomes a sharing community. It does not matter whether individual members are out distributing leaflets in the pubs, praying, talking to people in the club or washing up, we are all part of the body of Christ. Now, evening after evening, the team rallied round wielding scrubbing brushes, emulsion and gloss paint. Within a fortnight every door, wainscot and ceiling had been painted white.

One of the regular patrons of the club, hearing team members talk of my situation, offered his services as a paperhanger. Jimmy claimed to be a chef in one of the Edinburgh hotels; when tried, his recipes were very good. Something intangible in the man's face urged caution. I was sure that he had been in prison. I couldn't ask him; it wasn't the sort of question that could be asked. As he had been coming to the club longer than I had been in the team, I sought advice. The others did not think there was anything strange about him. If he had a criminal past, his presence in the club and his willingness to learn was probably a valiant attempt to put it all behind him. What right had I to judge?

During the General Assembly of the Church of Scotland that year, the new Moderator and other dignitaries visited Simon Square. They trouped past my desk where I was working on telephone accounts.

'And what happened to you?'

'Cerebral haemorrhage in '74.'

'Aren't you brave!'

'No, I had no alternative.'

I did not have the verbal ability to say it aloud so, while shaking hands, I said silently that all suffering, all disability, has to be shared if it is to be conquered. It has to be fought with rolled-up sleeves, learnt from, utilized. Only by sharing the dying person's fear of the unknown, the pain of the injured child, the hunger of the third world, can we begin to comprehend the suffering of God.

In the small office the Chaplain to the Lord High Commissioner had stood back to let the procession pass. He was watching me as I turned the palm of my left hand outwards, a method I had developed to enable me to shake hands without causing undue attention. I became aware that he was watching me and I looked up. He was a tall lean man whose face was lined with years of laughter. His eyes smiled warmly into mine, seeking to share the depths of my situation, the pain, the triumphs, the desolation. The smile was broadly returned. We looked at each other: he also had known much pain. Facing a man who was not afraid to accept the cost of sharing, it was as though someone had closed a door on the noise in the room. After the room had cleared, he came forward holding out his left hand. We talked for a few minutes and I was left with a profound sense of acceptance and peace.

The following week I was suddenly transferred to the Light Industrial Unit at Simon Square for assessment. On the first morning the Occupational Therapist covering the unit drew me aside. Along with the other social workers, I had been calling her Karen This was to stop; I was to call her Miss Baker. I was being put in my place. Trying to avoid sounding aggressive, I remarked that she must have a poor concept of her own ability or a superficial idea of professionalism if she needed to hide behind the protection of her surname. My task was to type lists of addresses onto envelopes. In that room, tasks were so simple and repetitive that most workers were unable to think beyond their next tea-break and their next cigarette. Only two of us worked consistently; progress was generally considered a mug's game.

The cottage was now almost unrecognizable. I felt uplifted

158

as help flooded in from friends realizing my dearth of essentials: lino for the kitchen and the hall, a chest of drawers, a chair, an electric fire. The floors had been scrubbed. Jimmy had decorated the bedroom and the hall, the kitchen and the sitting room. Now only the bathroom and the fourth wall in the sitting room remained. Tomorrow friends were coming to pack and transport small articles. Walking from room to room, I invited God to use the cottage for His purposes. I was the Lord's servant, so was my home. Surprisingly, I found myself thanking God for the privilege of being allowed to pay the rent. We both laughed. If I had seen the storm clouds gathering, it would have been much harder to make the same dedication.

When friends set off next day with the first two car loads of my belongings, I remained behind to organize the third load. They returned to report that when they had reached the cottage, a man had been waiting to help them unload, and was now wallpapering in the sitting room. Jimmy was the last person I wanted to know what was going in! Thank goodness silver and articles of value were either hidden at the bottom of boxes or else were coming with the carriers. When we arrived, Jimmy was finishing the fourth wall. I unloaded the case I would need again for the last journey tomorrow, carefully hiding my jewellery box underneath neat piles of clothes, and locked the drawer. Had I locked them all, the story might have been different.

On Monday the carriers agreed that I could travel with them. In the evening several friends arrived to help me unpack. Everything ran smoothly until I tried to open the chest of drawers. It moved slightly, then jammed. On closer inspection I found that somebody had removed the brass rim surrounding the keyhole. My heart-beat sounded like a drum in my ears. When we finally managed to open the drawer, the clothes were disordered and the box was sitting on top. Although my collection was small, it contained treasures which because of their family significance were irreplaceable. In the sitting room boxes had been ransacked of anything which the uneducated mind would conceive as having value.

It was the first of four robberies in ten days; the second and third happened on consecutive nights. After the third robbery, the police decided that entry was being made through the back door. They blocked it off and instructed the Corporation to change the locks. On the day after the first robbery I met Jane who invited me to return to the flat until my parents arrived the following Monday. They were coming up for their annual holiday. I felt very guilty about having to involve them in the inevitable turmoil and anxiety. They had planned to deliver my furniture and then we were to retreat into the Highlands for a much-needed rest.

It was as though both I and my values were being attacked, and not merely my property. I had begun so optimistically in faith; why was I being crushed? I knew that I had no right to ask, yet still the question came, 'Why?' A small voice inside my head said:

'If you retract the dedication, the robberies will stop.'

'No!'

I sat heavily on the temptation, squashing the life out of it. So that was it! The devil regarded the dedication as a threat and was retaliating. In fact the robberies were a twisted compliment. This would not be the end. With my refusal the devil would doubtless try again, but I knew that I would not be fighting in my own strength. God would hold me together.

I moved back into the cottage when my parents arrived a week later. The Police had arranged for the Post Office to move the telephone to my bedside. As the locks had been changed they thought that Jimmy would make another attempt at entry by breaking one of the rear windows. They planned that we would make the cottage appear empty, and lie in wait. For the next two nights, I dozed in bed with the rolling pin as a non-indictable defensive weapon beside me, as well as the front door keys to let the Police in, and my alarm clock muffled under the bedclothes. My father rested in an armchair in the hall and my mother sat, out of view, under the bedroom window.

On the third morning I became ill. It began with a headache; soon I had no speech, could neither stand nor grip anything, my vision was affected, I was getting blank patches in my hearing, and the colour had drained from my face. My mother telephoned my general practitioner who took one look at me and ordered an ambulance to which I was carried out on a stretcher. In Casualty I was put in a side-room and left. I was now vomiting bile. Although its acrid taste made me terribly thirsty, I immediately vomitted any water I drank. Pills automatically suffered the same fate. Eventually I was given an injection. Then a houseman arrived and announced that I could go home.

My mother read the exhaustion in my face and, in view of the response of the general practitioner, refused to move until I had been seen by a neurologist. My surgeon arrived during the evening and said that it was simply a migraine enlarged by stress. As it was getting late, the hospital kept me overnight before discharging me in the morning. In Casualty I was made to feel that I was there under false pretences, that I was attempting to cling to the hospital. When the ward heard about the robberies and the sleepless nights, they were very kind. By morning my head had cleared, my speech was very slowly returning but my legs were still very weak.

My parents had slept in their caravan overnight, and had returned to the cottage in the morning to discover the fourth robbery. The kitchen window had been broken, more property had been stolen, and there was a filthy mess. They refused to elaborate. They did not collect me until the afternoon because of clearing up and the police looking for fingerprints. Hospital staff wheeled me to the car but I was so unbalanced that I needed both my parents to help me down the front steps of the cottage. Yesterday's vomiting and inability to retain even sips of water had left me severely dehydrated. I sat listlessly in an armchair, scant tears wasting precious water, but without the energy even to cry. My speech had regressed a year; I was so low that I had no strength even to think clearly. My thoughts began and terminated in mid-sentence, leading nowhere. It was obvious that something would have to be done. My mother suggested that we all prayed. I confessed my failure, but reiterated the dedication. I might be weak, but God was not. That was the turning point. Later that evening my speech had almost returned to its previous level and I was able to enjoy a simple meal.

Early the following week, the police began to recover property. My father and I spent hours commuting between the Police Station and pawn shops, identifying and redeeming

161

possessions. While we were out, my mother cleaned and organized and cooked. My father also finished the decorating. They returned south physically and emotionally exhausted. The Detective Constable in charge of the case tried to reassure me:

'Don't you worry. He'll not bother you again. When we get him, he'll go down for a long time.'

They caught him with remarkable speed. He pleaded guilty, so he wasn't sent for trial but fined £50, approximately 5% of the value of the things stolen, and given time to pay. The police were furious.

CHAPTER TWENTY-TWO

No Compromise

The Occupational Therapists at the Cripple Aid Centre referred me to the Medical Adviser of the local Government Rehabilitation Centre. He was a large, rather bombastic man who listened somewhat superficially to what I said and propounded the great advantages of the Centre. He said that both industrial and clerical trades were available, and that they would teach me to type. I explained that during student vacations I had worked as a bi-lingual secretary in industry, and that as an out-patient I had converted my typing to the one-handed American method. Suddenly I had a brilliant idea. Could they teach me shorthand? I realized that it might mean a change in my field of employment but I did not want to waste my training. I wished to use my professional abilities to their fullest extent. The doctor replied that they could not teach me shorthand; they had no call for it.

He talked about the work. The day started at 7.45 a.m. so that workers could be introduced to a factory schedule. My assumption that clerical and professional workers started later was dispelled by the information that everyone started at the same time and that as a discouragement for late arrival, wages were cut. I did some mental calculations. I was now living at the other end of the city, between four and five miles away. The two bus journeys took an hour. Working steadily, it was taking me another hour to wash, dress and have breakfast. Could I get up at 5.45 a.m.? If I didn't, would other opportunities arise?

Having expended so much energy on achieving my present quality of survival, I realized that I was desperately afraid of stagnating. I could not face the possibility that progress or opportunity might suddenly cease. I asked the doctor whether I would be pushed into unstimulating work. His reply was condescending and evasive. I would begin on the construction of strawberry baskets to facilitate movement in my right hand. On my tour of the workfloor, I had watched them being made; it was extremely boring and repetitive work. I realized that it was not the intention that I end up a maker of strawberry baskets, but it set the level.

The doctor was expecting me to ask when I could begin. Instead I asked him whether his day started at 7.45 a.m. If it did, somehow I would manage the same. Greatly affronted, he spluttered that it did not. I shook my head: in that case, neither would mine. I would accept anything which made use of my professional abilities, but refused to be pushed along a path well below my capabilities. He was trying to force square pegs into round holes. Although it would have been interesting to gain experience of a government rehabilitation centre from the inside, the energy required would far outweigh the results achieved. Much to the doctor's surprise, I declined.

With the agreement of Simon Square, it had been arranged that I would spend July with my parents in England. It came as a thankful relief after the turmoil created by the robberies. When I got back to Edinburgh and reported to Simon Square, I was told that I was not to return, being considered too good for them. In collaboration with the Area Resettlement Adviser from the Employment Service Agency, I was referred to an Occupational Psychologist. I leapt at the chance; he would be able to give guidance about what would be realistic yet interesting work.

Mr King was a quiet man, prepared to consider my aptitudes, personality and experience. We related well and had five lengthy meetings during September and October. He did an extensive range of tests and was surprised by the interest I showed in the technical side of my assessment. Although my manual dexterity was limited by the paralysis, extensive compensation was provided by my left hand. Had I ever thought of becoming an artist? I said that in hospital I had briefly toyed with the idea, but had no formal training except O-level Art. He thought my linguistic usage and ability to conceptualize were good. Major brain surgery had foreshortened my short-term memory, but I was automatically developing self-prompting techniques.

164

He finished his assessment. I was suitable either for social work administration, or postgraduate librarianship which would require further training. I was surprised; I had always visualized myself working among people rather than books. Financing further training could prove difficult, so we settled on social work administration. He expected me to return later to direct practice, but regretted that he would be unable to help me find a post. He would now forward his report to the Disablement Resettlement Officer. I now had his professional confirmation that a return to social work would not be an unrealistic dream.

During the summer of 1976, I became the representative of the British Association of Social Workers on the Scottish Council on Disability. Later I also became a founder member of the Scottish Committee on Mobility for the Disabled. My responsibility in representing both the social work profession and clients on these voluntary committees served to maintain my determination to gain employment in a setting in which my experience could be well used. At regular intervals I received circulars from the Job Centre saying that they had not received notification of any suitable posts. They asked me for information about any change in circumstance, promising a stamped addressed envelope. It was never enclosed, possibly as a deterrent to my reply.

Still unemployed in May 1977, despite eighteen months of applications, a post was advertised which was so directly relevant that it seemed too good to be true. It was a joint appointment between Edinburgh University and the Social Work Department to undertake research entitled 'Education for Disability'. But could I manage? There was bound to be some teaching later on. Would my speech stand up it it? I submitted an application, and was interviewed by a board of five. Questions and answers were rapidly, positively and extensively exchanged for three-quarters of an hour. I came out feeling elated. I did not get the job, but that interview re-affirmed my sense of professional self-worth.

I submitted applications whenever relevant opportunities arose. They were met either by silence or rejection. Nobody wanted to risk being first to employ me. Everyone wanted to share in the triumph represented by my survival, but few had the courage to help with my rehabilitation. Was I wrong in trying to return to the work for which I had been trained? Too often employers avoid coming to terms with their own fears about disability by persistently underestimating the potential of disabled employees. I had withstood pressure to acknowledge relegation by society, not from inability to accept the concept of another job, but from acute awareness of the wastage of skill and years of government money.

Perhaps I should give up and take any post? As a Christian, did it matter what job I had? I would still belong to God and still serve Him. However, my capitulation would be negative collusion. The disabled have little choice in the identity they create: they are pushed by society into the identity of their disability. It is not so much the experience of disablement which destroys the individual, but the public response. I faced my fears and my limited sphere of influence. The choice between principle and expediency always remains: if I gave in, all society would learn was that another disabled person had failed in her bid for rehabilitation. Yet I had no right to give up; it was not just me living, but Christ living in me.

From my earliest days in the cottage, I had decided that it should be a place where friends would always be welcome. Sometimes several of them came to dinner, filling the place with laughter. Only too pleased of the company, I said nothing about the limitations imposed by feeding a group from a benefit intended for one. When I was about to run out of something important, a food parcel would arrive from my mother. The timing of their arrival was uncanny. When the store cupboard and my benefit were low it was God who, with unfailing precision, inspired unwitting friends to invite me for meals.

Bills have the unfortunate habit of arriving in convoy. The gas bill devoured three weeks' money. Almost a month's income disappeared into the electricity bill and maintenance for my washing machine. I had eaten my way through the contents of the freezer and reduced the standard of my diet. The telephone bill was imminent. There were no parcels, no invitations. Struggling against dejection, the situation permeated every corner of my existence, dominating my prayer life. I was chided by Luther: 'What more can the devil do than slay us? Why worry then, since Christ is at the helm?' I could trust God for the future from the example of everything He had done in the past.

One afternoon there was a knock at the door. It was a young boy from the local primary school. He handed me two bags of shopping as a present from the children in his class. It must have taken days to organize. The thoughtfulness of those children and their teacher and the gentle, chiding reassurance of God were overwhelming. 'Give and it will be given unto you; good measure, pressed down, shaken together, running over will be put into your lap.' I hugged the boy, tears of gratitude and relief running down my face. Astounded, he beat a hasty retreat.

Summer came and went. In late autumn 1977, Lothian Region announced the inauguration of a register of locum hospital social workers. I applied and was interviewed by the Principal Social Worker from the city's children's hospital. She became the first social worker to recognize, in an interview, my positive integration of professional experience and personal history. Her perception and lack of defence were a pleasure to encounter. After two further interviews, I was appointed in January 1978 to a three-month locum post in a hospital some miles from Edinburgh. The task was to assess and quantify the need for social work input within a hospital unit caring for 112 long-stay patients. It was the coldest winter for two hundred years. I stayed in the nurses' home three nights a week, having agreed to complete five days' work in four days. Amongst all the ice and snow, I felt an indescribable lightness of heart. Aware that my performance was being closely monitored, I worked consistently and with great energy. Despite the success of this post, subsequent applications were rejected.

When this book was begun, I could hardly put two sentences together. Now, five years later, I am writing fluently and, apart from the occasional dyspraxic mistake, my speech is normal. Why should the extent and quality of my survival have been so profound? My progress stems from the knowledge that I am not my own, but Christ's. I knew that from the mustard seed of my faith, God could create a tree. In the context of His strength, my vulnerability and the ridicule of an agnostic public become irrelevant. The struggle continues, but in Christ its heart is peace. This book is a tribute to the small group of people who had the courage to share in the vision of survival and rehabilitation. It is a testimony not to the strength of man, but to the wisdom, power and infinite love of God.